Handbook of Dietary Supplements

Vitamins and other Health Supplements

D0588390

Also of interest:

NUTRITION AND DIETARY ADVICE
IN THE PHARMACY
Pamela Mason
0–632–03427–0

MANUAL OF DIETETIC PRACTICE
Second Edition
Edited by Briony Thomas
0–632–03003–8

OTC MEDICATIONS
*Symptoms and treatments of
common illnesses*
Second Edition
A. Li Wan Po
G. Li Wan Po
0–632–04046–7

SYMPTOMS IN THE PHARMACY
Second Edition
A. Blenkinsopp and P. Paxton
0–632–03609–5

STATISTICS FOR PHARMACISTS
A. Li Wan Po
0–632–04881–6

 NON-PRESCRIPTION DRUGS
Second Edition
A. Li Wan Po
0–632–02672–3

PHARMACY LAW AND PRACTICE
Second Edition
Jonathan Merrills and Jonathan Fisher
0–632–03232–4

NUTRITION IN PRIMARY CARE
Briony Thomas
0–632–03981–7

Handbook of Dietary Supplements

Vitamins and other Health Supplements

PAMELA MASON
BSc, MSc, PhD, MRPharmS

Blackwell
Science

© 1995 by
Blackwell Science Ltd
Editorial Offices:
Osney Mead, Oxford OX2 0EL
25 John Street, London WC1N 2BL
23 Ainslie Place, Edinburgh EH3 6AJ
350 Main Street, Malden
 MA 02148 5018, USA
54 University Street, Carlton
 Victoria 3053, Australia
10, rue Casimir Delavigne
 75006 Paris, France

Other Editorial Offices:

Blackwell Wissenschafts-Verlag GmbH
Kurfürstendamm 57
10707 Berlin, Germany

Blackwell Science KK
MG Kodenmacho Building
7–10 Kodenmacho Nihombashi
Chuo-ku, Tokyo 104, Japan

The right of the Author to be identified as the
Author of this Work has been asserted in
accordance with the Copyright, Designs and
Patents Act 1988.

All rights reserved. No part of this publication may
be reproduced, stored in a retrieval system, or
transmitted, in any form or by any means,
electronic, mechanical, photocopying, recording
or otherwise, except as permitted by the UK
Copyright, Designs and Patents Act 1988,
without the prior permission of the publisher.

First published 1995
Reprinted 1998

Set by DP Photosetting, Aylesbury, Bucks
Printed and bound in Great Britain by
MPG Books Ltd, Bodmin, Cornwall

The Blackwell Science logo is a
trade mark of Blackwell Science Ltd,
registered at the United Kingdom
Trade Marks Registry

DISTRIBUTORS

Marston Book Services Ltd
PO Box 269
Abingdon
Oxon OX14 4YN
(Orders: Tel: 01235 465500
         Fax: 01235 465555)

USA
Blackwell Science, Inc.
Commerce Place
350 Main Street
Malden, MA 02148 5018
(Orders: Tel: 800 759 6102
              781 388 8250
         Fax: 781 388 8255)

Canada
Login Brothers Book Company
324 Saulteaux Crescent
Winnipeg, Manitoba R3J 3T2
(Orders: Tel: 204 224 4068)

Australia
Blackwell Science Pty Ltd
54 University Street
Carlton, Victoria 3053
(Orders: Tel: 03 9347 0300
         Fax: 03 9347 5001)

A catalogue record for this title
is available from the British Library

ISBN 0-632-03923-X

Library of Congress
Cataloging in Publication Data
is available

Contents

Preface

More than a third of the UK population supplement their daily diet with vitamins and health supplements and, in Britain, over £200 million is spent each year on these products.

Health professionals, including pharmacists, dietitians, general practitioners, practice nurses and health visitors are frequently asked for advice about supplements, but they often have difficulty in finding the necessary information to help them give rational advice. And because there can be few areas of healthcare where so many misconceptions and so much confusion exists, the need for a source of sound, unbiased advice about supplements is overwhelming. This book has been written to help health professionals to give such advice.

In preparing this book, I have attempted to make the information accessible and easy to use. Supplements are arranged by generic name in alphabetical order and information is given, where appropriate, under the same standard headings throughout. Information about the majority of the dietary supplement products available on the UK market, together with the names and addresses of manufacturers, and a detailed index are provided at the end of the book. It is not intended to be a textbook on vitamins.

This handbook will help health professionals to:

- recognize groups of people who could benefit from supplements,
- distinguish between scientifically accepted and controversial uses for supplements,
- advise on dietary sources of vitamins and minerals,
- ask patients appropriate questions about supplement use,
- recommend appropriate products and correct doses,
- identify individuals for whom specific supplements could be contra-indicated,
- recognize the risk for adverse effects from supplement misuse,
- identify supplements which may interact with drugs and vice versa, and
- identify supplements which may interfere with laboratory test values.

Acknowledgements are due to the many manufacturers of dietary supplements who provided information about their products for this handbook. I would also like to thank colleagues at the Royal Pharmaceutical Society and the National Pharmaceutical Association for their advice and friendship while the book was being written, and my husband, Ambrose, and my mother for their continuing support and encouragement.

Pamela Mason

Chapter 1
How to use this book

This book covers 54 commonly available dietary supplements, including vitamins, minerals, trace elements, antioxidants and other substances, such as garlic, ginseng and fish oils. For ease of reference, they are arranged in alphabetical order and give information, where appropriate, under the following standard headings:

Description
States the type of substance; e.g. a vitamin, mineral, enzyme, plant extract etc.

Nomenclature
Lists names and alternative names in current usage. Definitions of names for vitamins were obtained from: Nomenclature Policy: Generic Descriptors and Trivial Names for Vitamins and Related Compounds. *J Nutr* **117**, 7–14. Alternative names for some substances were obtained from Martindale, *The Extra Pharmacopoeia*, 30th edition (1993).

Units
Includes alternative units and conversion factors.

Constituents
Lists active ingredients in supplements that are not pure vitamins or minerals (e.g. evening primrose oil contains gamma-linolenic acid).

Human requirements
Lists UK Dietary Reference Values for different ages and sex. These figures were obtained (and used with permission) from The Department of Health's *Dietary Reference Values for Food Energy and Nutrients for the United Kingdom* (1991).

Intakes
States amounts of nutrients provided by the average adult diet in the UK. Figures were obtained from: Bull & Buss (1982); Bunker *et al.* (1984); Bunker *et al.* (1988a) and (1988b); Gregory *et al.* (1990); Spring *et al.* (1979); Tsongas *et al.* (1980); Wenlock *et al.* (1979).

Action
Explains the role of the substance in maintaining bodily function and pharmacological actions where appropriate.

Dietary sources

Lists significant food sources based on average portion sizes. Tables used as sources (with permission) for figures include: *McCance and Widdowson's The Composition of Foods* (1991) and Davies & Dickerson's *Nutrient Content of Food Portions* (1991).

In addition, a food may be described as an **excellent** or *good* source of a nutrient. This does not describe any food as 'excellent' or 'good' overall. It defines only the amount of the nutrient (per portion or serving) in relation to the Reference Nutrient Intake (RNI) of the nutrient for the average adult male. Thus, an excellent source provides 50% or more of the RNI and a good source provides 15–50% of the RNI. Where no RNI has been set for a particular nutrient, **excellent** and *good* are numerically defined.

Metabolism

Discusses absorption, transport, distribution and excretion.

Bioavailability

Includes the effects of cooking, processing, storage methods, and substances in food which may alter bioavailability.

Deficiency

Lists signs and symptoms of deficiency.

Uses

Emphasis is given to the use of the substance as a dietary supplement and discussion of the controversial claims made. Medically recognized indications for vitamins and minerals are summarized in Section 59, Appendix 3.

Precautions/contra-indications

Lists diseases and conditions in which the substance should be avoided or used with caution.

Pregnancy and breast-feeding

Comments on safety or potential toxicity during pregnancy and lactation.

Adverse effects

Describes the risks that may accompany excessive intake, and signs and symptoms of toxicity.

Interactions

Lists drugs and other nutrients which may interact with the supplement. This includes drugs that affect vitamin and mineral status and supplements which influence drug metabolism.

Interference with diagnostic tests

Vitamins, minerals and supplements may increase or decrease laboratory values for other substances measured in body fluids (resulting in false positive or false negative tests).

Dose
> Gives dosage range present in available supplements. The British National Formulary or company data sheets should be consulted for doses of vitamins and minerals in clinical use.

References and/or further reading
> A list of those cited in the text and sometimes sources of further information. In addition there are the following appendixes.

Products
> Section 57, appendix 1, which lists products generically in the same order as the main entries; multiple-ingredient products are tabulated separately.

Medically recognized indications for vitamins and minerals
> Section 58, Appendix 2, which summarizes the main prescribable (by doctors) indications for vitamins and minerals. Supplements should not be sold over the counter for the indications in Appendix 2.

Directory of manufacturers
> Section 59, Appendix 3, which gives names, addresses, telephone and facsimile numbers of product manufacturers.

References

Bull N.L. & Buss D.H. (1982) Biotin, pantothenic acid and vitamin E in the British household food supply. *Hum Nutr: Appl Nutr* **36A**, 190–6.

Bunker V.W., Lawson M.S., Delves H.T. & Clayton B.E. (1984) The uptake and excretion of chromium by the elderly. *Am J Clin Nutr* **39**, 797–802.

Bunker V.W., Lawson M.S., Stansfield M.F. & Clayton B.E. (1988a) Selenium balance studies in apparently healthy and housebound people eating self-selected diets. *Br J Nutr* **59**, 171–80.

Bunker V.W., Lawson M.S., Stansfield M.F. & Clayton B.E. (1988b) Trace element nutrition in the elderly – a review of zinc, copper, manganese and chromium. *Int Clin Nutr Rev* **8**, 111–27.

Davies J. & Dickerson J. (1991) *Nutrient Content of Food Portions*. The Royal Society of Chemistry, Cambridge.

Gregory J., Foster K., Tyler H. & Wiseman M. (1990) *The dietary and nutritional survey of British adults*. HMSO, London.

Holland B., Welch A.A., Unwin I.D., Buss D.H., Paul A.A. & Southgate D.A.T. (1991) *McCance and Widdowson's The Composition of Foods* 5th edn. The Royal Society of Chemistry and Ministry of Agriculture, Fisheries and Food, London.

Spring J.A., Robertson J. & Buss D.H. (1979) Trace nutrients 3: Magnesium, copper, zinc, vitamin B_6, vitamin B_{12}, and folic acid in the British household food supply. *Br J Nutr* **41**, 487–93.

Tsongas T.A., Meglen R.R., Walravens P.A. & Chappell W.R. (1980) Molybdenum in the diet: an estimate of average intakes in the United States. *Am J Clin Nutr* **33**, 1103–7.

Wenlock R.W., Buss D.H. & Dixon E.J. (1979) Trace elements 2: Manganese in British diets. *Br J Nutr* **41**, 253–61.

Chapter 2
Introduction

There is now considerable interest in dietary supplements and the public are increasingly asking questions about them. Thirty five per cent of adults regularly use these products and, in the UK in 1993, sales of dietary supplements were £238 million (Benn Publications, 1994).

While there is a great deal of information about these substances, not all of it is reliable. Indeed, there are probably few areas associated with healthcare where such confusion exists.

This confusion extends to health professionals as well as the general public. Because dietary supplements are not considered to be drugs, pharmacists are often unfamiliar with them and because they are not foods (in the sense of being part of a normal diet) dietitians are, understandably, wary of recommending them. Doctors typically receive little nutritional education and may not have the knowledge to give informed advice.

In addition, supplements are a topic about which there is a great deal of disagreement even between nutrition experts. Some say they are largely unnecessary because a balanced diet provides all the required vitamins and minerals, while others say that supplements make a worthwhile contribution to a healthy diet.

What are dietary supplements?

Definition

For the purposes of this book, dietary supplements are defined as products which contain vitamins, minerals and/or other ingredients, such as fish oils and ginseng, which consumers believe to be beneficial for their health. They are normally sold in the form of tablets, capsules, powders or liquids. Under EC law, they are known as 'diet integrators'.

Enteral feeds (e.g. Complan and Ensure) and slimming aids are also classified as dietary supplements by nutritionists and dietitians, but for the purposes of this book these products will be ignored.

Classification

Dietary supplements fall into several categories.

1. Vitamins and minerals
   (a) Multi-vitamins and minerals, which normally contain around 100% of the Reference Nutrient Intake (RNI) for vitamins, with varying amounts of minerals and trace elements.
   (b) Single vitamins and minerals, which often contain very large amounts. When levels exceed ten times the RNI, they are termed 'megadoses'.

(c) Combinations of vitamins and minerals, marketed for specific population groups e.g. athletes, children, pregnant women, slimmers, teenagers, vegetarians etc.

(d) Combinations of vitamins and minerals with other substances, such as evening primrose oil and ginseng.

2. 'Unofficial' vitamins and minerals, for which a requirement and a deficiency disorder in humans has not, so far, been recognized, e.g. choline, inositol, germanium, silicon.

3. Natural oils containing fatty acids for which there is some evidence of beneficial effects, e.g. evening primrose oil and fish oils.

4. Natural substances containing ingredients with recognized pharmacological actions but whose composition and effects have not been fully defined, e.g. garlic, ginkgo biloba and ginseng.

5. Natural substances whose composition and effects are not well defined but which are marketed for their 'health giving properties', e.g. chlorella, royal jelly and spirulina.

6. Enzymes with known physiological effects, but of doubtful efficacy when taken by mouth e.g. superoxide dismutase.

Legal status

Some vitamin and mineral products are licensed medicines (e.g. Abidec drops and Pregaday tablets) and some, but not all, of these are prescribable on the NHS. A few preparations containing gamma-linolenic acid (e.g. Epogam and Efamast) and fish oil (e.g. Maxepa) are also prescribable on the NHS. However, the majority of supplements are classified legally as foods.

Unlike medicines, most supplements are not, therefore, subject to the controls of the Medicines Act 1968. Because supplements classed as foods do not require product licences, they do not have to go through clinical trials, and are therefore much cheaper to put on the market than medicines.

Dietary supplements are not controlled by the same strict conditions of dosage, labelling, purity criteria and levels of ingredients as medicines. Concern about this relative lack of regulation has been expressed and some recommendations have been published by the World Health Organisation Regional Office for Europe (1993). The retail supply of those vitamins which have product licences (i.e. medicines) is subject to limitations which depend on the product's strength and maximum daily dose as shown in Table 2.1.

Vitamin products which are legally classified as foods are not subject to such limitations, and dietary supplements containing levels of vitamins in excess of those in prescription only medicines are easily available to the public. For example, it is possible to buy supplements containing 7.5 mg (25 000 units) of vitamin A in a single dose.

Quality assurance

Purity standards for dietary supplements are not quite so exacting as they are for medicines. Medicines are subject to rigorous quality control, including disintegration and bioavailability tests, and precision as to levels of ingredients and contaminants.

Table 2.1 Limitations on the sale or supply of licensed medicines containing certain vitamins

Vitamin	Legal status
Vitamin A	Up to 2250 μg (7 500 units) **GSL** Over 2250 μg (7 500 units) **POM**
Vitamin D	Up to 10 μg (400 units) **GSL** Over 10 μg (400 units) **P**
Cyanocobalamin	Up to 10 μg **GSL** Over 10 μg **P**
Folic acid	Up to 200 μg **GSL** 200–500 μg **P** Over 500 μg **POM**

GSL: subject to control under the Medicines (General Sales List) Order 1977
POM: subject to control under the Medicines (Prescriptions Only) Order 1977
P: Pharmacy only products

There is some evidence that amounts of vitamins and minerals in food supplements vary somewhat from levels stated on product labels. For example, a report in *Which? Way to Health* (1994) demonstrated some differences between the gamma-linolenic acid content of evening primrose oil supplements and the amounts declared on labels. In addition, contaminants, including arsenic, cadmium, lead and mercury have been found in supplements such as bonemeal (see Section 6), dolomite (see Section 17) and kelp (see Section 31).

Labels

Supplements which are foods are subject to the Food Labelling Regulations 1984, while those that are medicines must be labelled according to the provisions of the Medicines Act. The Food Labelling Regulations require a full list of ingredients, both active and inactive, on the label. Excipients, such as gluten and lactose must be included. The Medicines Act originally required that only active ingredients must be listed. Since January 1994, however, all new products and older products with renewed product licences must be labelled with all ingredients, including excipients.

However, the amounts of vitamins and minerals found in food supplements may not be an entirely accurate reflection of the strengths stated on labels. Quantities of drugs declared on medicine labels fall within agreed standards, usually those of the British Pharmacopoeia.

Supplement labels may be extremely confusing to the public. For example, different manufacturers use different types of unit to express nutrient content; some use international units, others micrograms and milligrams. And, in accordance with the Food Labelling Regulations, supplement labels are normally expressed in terms of Recommended Daily Amounts (RDA) rather than the more recent term, Reference Nutrient Intakes (RNI). When RDAs are used on supplement labels, they usually take the following form:

one tablet (or daily dose) of the supplement provides x% of the RDA for vitamin (or mineral) y.

Nutrition labelling is to be standardized throughout Europe and an EC Directive came into operation in October 1993. However, food supplements are exempt from this directive and a later directive is likely to specify labelling requirements for these products.

The strength of some products is stated in terms of the substance used rather than the nutrient, for example calcium carbonate rather than calcium, evening primrose oil rather than gamma-linolenic acid, fish oil rather than omega-3 fatty acids. This makes it difficult to compare products.

Claims

Dietary supplements are vigorously promoted, but unlike licensed medicines, they may not be promoted for medicinal use. No claim may be made that a dietary supplement is capable of curing, treating or preventing human disease. Wording such as 'this product prevents heart disease' or 'this product lowers blood pressure' is illegal and constitutes an offence.

Despite this prohibition, the potential for supplements to mislead the public is enormous. This is often more a matter of what is implied than what is actually said. Wording such as 'this product may help to reduce blood cholesterol" may be interpreted by consumers to mean that such a product will definitely prevent heart attacks.

Claims such as 'this product can help to maintain good health at the time of the menopause' or 'many people report improved energy levels with this product' or 'maintains the health of the circulation' constitute health claims; these are allowed. Health claims are not allowed to name diseases, but they may refer to possible disease risk factors (e.g. blood cholesterol) and also to body organs or systems.

Most members of the public are not in a position to distinguish between the different types of claims or to discern their truthfulness. All too often, the overall impression given by advertisements is that we are all on the verge of nutritional deficiency due to stress, environmental pollutants and processed foods so the best solution is to take a supplement.

One of the most popular themes of advertising is related to stress and its effects on vitamin requirements. This has resulted in a plethora of stress formulas. Stress, however, is never properly defined. While injury, infection, fever, shock, illness and surgery can certainly increase nutrient requirements, there is little scientific evidence that the stress of everyday life increases the risk of deficiency, unless that stress results in the consumption of a poor diet for an extended period of time.

While the level of misinformation associated with supplements is no greater than that attached to many other products (e.g. cosmetics and household cleaners), the risk to health is increased if supplements are misused. This is not generally true of cosmetics. Consumers should be discouraged from using excessive doses of supplements which could be harmful, and from using such products in the place of more orthodox disease treatment, particularly without the knowledge of their doctor.

Evidence for claims

So-called 'evidence' for claims made for supplements is often scanty, conflicting and inconclusive and based on uncontrolled clinical trials or anecdotal reports. Only a few supplement ingredients have been subjected to extensive scientific evaluation to determine the validity of their role in disease prevention or treatment.

In order to provide evidence that a specific vitamin or mineral prevents disease, for example, four questions need to be answered:

1. Is there evidence for an inverse relationship between blood and/or tissue levels of a vitamin or mineral and risk of disease?

2. What blood levels of the vitamin or mineral are required to reduce the risk of disease?

3. Is there evidence for an inverse relationship between intake of the vitamin or mineral and risk of disease?

4. What level of intake of the vitamin or mineral is required to reduce the risk of disease?

Three types of trials (all double-blind) are needed to provide evidence that an increased level of a vitamin or mineral will reduce the risk of disease:

1. A cross-cultural epidemiological study must show that there is a statistically proven association between low levels of intake of a nutrient in a sample population, demonstrated by low plasma levels of that nutrient, and high risk of disease.

2. Prospective trials must show that there is a correlation between a low initial serum level of the nutrient and high subsequent risk of the disease in individuals in the same study group.

3. Intervention trials must show that a supplement of the nutrient to the diet of a sample population then leads, in the absence of any other intervention, to a reduced incidence of the disease as compared to a similar group to whom only a placebo is administered.

Only when evidence has been obtained from all three types of study can it be said with certainty that a supplement will be effective. For some supplements (e.g. antioxidants) there is some evidence available from epidemiological studies, but very little from intervention studies. Claims for others, as has been mentioned already, rely on anecdote, animal studies only or single case studies.

Natural versus synthetic

Of the multitude of claims made for supplements, 'natural' is probably one of the most emotive; natural products are believed to be safer than synthetic ones and also more efficacious. Yet the body cannot distinguish between a vitamin molecule derived from a synthetic source and one derived from a natural source; both are absorbed and used, with some exceptions (e.g. vitamin E), in the same way. Synthetic vitamins are also generally much less expensive than 'natural' vitamins.

Whether a vitamin product is natural or synthetic is open to debate. The usual understanding of natural supplements is that they are those whose active ingredients were present in the original source material (e.g. vitamin C concentrated from rosehips or acerola cherries), while synthetic supplements are those whose active ingredients are manufactured by chemical synthesis from non-nutrient precursors (e.g. vitamin A synthesized from acetylene or beta-ionone).

However, 'natural' products may not be quite as natural as consumers think. Levels of 'natural' vitamin C in a supplement may be increased by the addition of vitamin C made in a laboratory. Extraction of vitamins from natural sources (e.g. vitamin B from yeast or vitamin E from vegetable oils) normally involves the use of a number of laboratory processes.

One of the arguments used in favour of natural vitamins is that vitamins tend to occur in nature in combination with synergistic factors (e.g. vitamin C with bioflavonoids), whereas synthetic vitamins are not associated with such factors. But synthetic products are also devoid of inhibitory factors, such as oxalic acid and phytic acid, which tend to form complexes with vitamins and minerals in nature.

Patterns of supplement use

More than one third of the UK population buy dietary supplements and of these 70% are women, mostly between the ages of 35 and 65. Individuals with professional occupations buy more supplements than manual workers.

Sales of some of the different types of supplements (1993 figures) are shown in Table 2.2.

Table 2.2 Sales of different types of supplements in the UK (1993 figures)

Total	£238m
Fish oils	£66m
Multivitamins	£62m
Single vitamins	£35m
Evening primrose oil and other GLA products	£35m
Garlic	£21m
Other	£19m

GLA: Gamma-linolenic acid.
Source: Benn Publications (1994) *The OTC Healthcare Report*

In 1993 pharmacies sold just over half of all the supplements in the UK, with Boots accounting for 35%. Grocers sold just under one third of the total, drugstores 14% and healthfood stores 12%.

Reasons for supplement use

Reasons for buying supplements are many and varied and may include the following:

- as an insurance policy to supplement what an individual may consider to be a poor diet (e.g. no time or inclination to eat regular meals),
- to improve overall health and fitness,
- to prolong vitality and delay the onset of age-associated problems,
- as a tonic or 'pick-me-up' when feeling run-down or after illness,
- for stress,

- recommended by an alternative health practitioner or health professional,
- pregnancy,
- slimming,
- smoking,
- to improve performance and body building in sports and athletics,
- to prevent or treat various signs and symptoms (e.g. colds, high blood cholesterol, poor sight, skin problems, arthritis, pre-menstrual syndrome etc.), or
- to improve children's IQ.

Use of supplements may be quite legitimate and, in order to understand who might benefit from them, it is important to have some appreciation of how nutrient requirements are assessed – in other words, what is meant by dietary standards and how they are established.

Dietary standards

Historical perspective

The isolation and identification of vitamins occurred in the first half of the 20th century between 1900 and 1948. The association of specific diseases with deficiency of certain vitamins (e.g. scurvy with deficiency of vitamin C, niacin with pellagra etc.) led to the development of 'standards' against which people's nutrient intakes could be measured.

Such standards have existed in the UK for nearly 40 years. The most recent standards have been in the form of Recommended Intakes of nutrients (DHSS 1969), Recommended Daily Amounts of food energy and nutrients (DHSS 1979) and Dietary Reference Values (DoH 1991).

Nutrient requirements vary according to age, sex and physiological status (e.g. pregnancy and lactation) and figures are provided for males and females in specific age ranges and also for pregnant and lactating women. The number of nutrients included in the standards continually increases and can be expected to increase further in the future as more information becomes available.

Recommended Daily Amounts

Most health professionals will be familiar with the term 'Recommended Daily Amount' (RDA) for vitamins and minerals. RDA is the standard used on the labels of dietary supplements.

The problem with RDAs is that they are much misused. The term 'recommended' means that some people attribute a greater degree of accuracy to these figures than was ever intended.

All too often the RDA is interpreted as the minimum desirable intake for optimal health and an amount which everybody must consume. In reality, the RDA covers the needs of most of the population, even those with high requirements, and is in excess of what most individuals require. RDAs were never intended to be used by individuals to assess their diets.

Dietary Reference Values

Dietary Reference Values (DRVs) are the most recent UK dietary standards.

These have been developed in an attempt to overcome the misuse of RDAs. Thus, the term 'recommended' has been replaced by 'reference' to emphasize the true nature of the figures which are estimates or reference values and not absolute recommendations for intakes by individuals.

In addition, a single figure, the RDA, has been replaced by several (see Table 2.3). This should also reduce the potential for misuse. These new figures, like the old RDAs, are based on the assumption that the requirements for nutrients in a population follow a normal distribution curve (see Figure 2.1). The Estimated Average Requirement (EAR) is the mean requirement; the Reference Nutrient Intake (RNI) is, like the old RDA, set at two standard deviations above the mean, and the Lower Reference Nutrient Intake (LRNI) at two standard deviations below the mean.

Table 2.3 Definition of dietary standards

DRV	*Dietary Reference Value.* A term used to cover LRNI, EAR, RNI and Safe Intake.
EAR	*Estimated Average Requirement.* An assessment of the average requirement for energy or protein or a vitamin or mineral. About half the population will need more than the EAR, and half less.
LRNI	*Lower Reference Nutrient Intake.* The amount of protein, vitamin or mineral which is considered to be sufficient for the few people in a group who have low needs. Most people will need more than the LRNI and if people consistently consume less they may be at risk of deficiency of that nutrient.
RNI	*Reference Nutrient Intake.* The amount of protein, vitamin or mineral which is sufficient for almost every individual. This level of intake is much higher than many people need.
	Safe Intake. A term used to indicate an intake or range of intakes of a nutrient for which there is not enough information to estimate the RNI, EAR or LRNI. It is considered to be adequate for almost everyone's needs but not large enough to cause undesirable effects.
RDA	*Recommended Daily Amount.* The average amount of energy or a nutrient recommended to cover the needs of groups of healthy people.

Estimation of dietary standards

Dietary standards are developed from a knowledge of nutrient requirements. The problem is that nutrient requirements cannot be accurately measured. They can only be estimated. A combination of reliable experimental data, epidemiological associations and even anecdotal data may be used for this purpose.

Information used to estimate requirements includes:

- the intake of a nutrient required to prevent or cure clinical signs of deficiency,
- the intake of a nutrient required to maintain balance (i.e. intake – output = zero),
- the intake of a nutrient required to maintain a given blood level, tissue concentration or degree of enzyme saturation, and
- the intake of a nutrient in the diet of a healthy population.

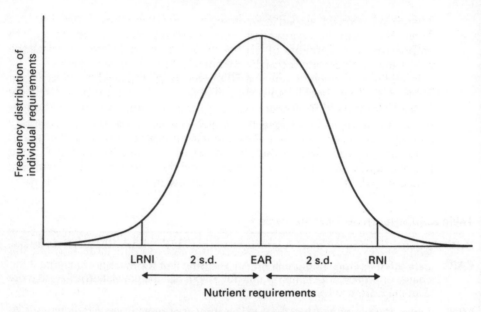

Figure 2.1 Frequency distribution of nutrient requirements

It is impossible to produce accurate figures for dietary requirements using such criteria, but they are the only criteria currently available.

Uses of dietary standards

Appropriate uses of dietary standards include:

- the evaluation of the adequacy of the national food supply,
- the establishment of standards for institutional meal planning,
- the establishment of nutritional policy for all institutions e.g. hospitals,
- the evaluation of diets in food consumption studies,
- the development of materials for nutrition education,
- the establishment of labelling regulations, and
- the development of guidelines for food product formulation.

Limitations of dietary standards

The fact that dietary standards should not be used to assess the diets of individuals has been mentioned already. Dietary standards do not give ideal or optimum intakes for individuals. People differ from each other in the amounts of nutrients they need and the quantities they absorb and utilize.

The imprecision in estimating both dietary standards and a person's nutrient intake means that utmost caution must be used in applying the figures to individuals. At best, they can give no more than a guide to the adequacy of a person's diet.

So, for example, if an individual is typically consuming the RNI for a particular nutrient, it can be assumed that his or her diet provides adequate amounts (or more than adequate amounts) of that nutrient. But if intake is regularly below the RNI, it cannot necessarily be assumed that the diet is inadequate, because that person may have a lower requirement for that nutrient.

However, if an individual is consistently consuming less than the LRNI for a nutrient, it can be assumed that the diet is deficient in that nutrient.

In addition, dietary standards apply only to healthy people, and not to those with disease whose nutrient needs may be very different. Requirements may be increased:

- in patients with disorders of the gastro-intestinal tract, liver and kidney,
- in those with inborn errors of metabolism, cancer, AIDS, severe infections, wounds or burns, and
- following surgery.

Drug administration may also alter nutrient requirements.

Future perspectives

Dietary standards have traditionally been based on the amounts of nutrients required to prevent deficiency disease. It is not too difficult to find out the amount of vitamin C that will prevent scurvy. But is prevention of deficiency signs enough? Would larger amounts of nutrients confer benefits beyond the prevention of deficiency?

Evidence is increasing that, in addition to prevention of deficiency disorders, most essential nutrients have a variety of physiological effects at different levels of intake. For example, vitamin E in amounts larger than the RNI appears to protect against cancer and coronary heart disease. It is therefore possible that nutrients could influence the development of a variety of diseases when ingested in quantities larger than the RNI.

While there is agreement about the beneficial effects of nutrients in the prevention of deficiency disease and the amounts required to achieve such effects, there is enormous controversy about amounts required for so-called 'optimum health'. Some would argue that higher amounts are required and that basing requirements for nutrients only on the prevention of deficiency disease is inadequate. But what other end points should be used is open to debate: longevity, increased resistance to cancer and coronary heart disease, improved athletic performance?

One of the problems with increasing the figures is that higher levels of intake cannot always easily be obtained from the diet alone – supplementation is required. In addition, excessive intake of some nutrients can lead to toxicity. While evidence is accumulating for beneficial effects of certain nutrients at levels of intake above the RNI, further studies are required to confirm such effects.

If dosage is increased beyond the physiological range, no further physiological effect is expected, but pharmacological actions may occur. Such pharmacological effects may have little to do with the physiological importance of the nutrient. For example, nicotinic acid, at 200 times the RNI, lowers serum cholesterol and triglycerides – a pharmacological response.

Who needs supplements?

The traditional answer to this question is that a 'balanced diet' supplies all the necessary nutrients and that supplements are required only for the treatment of established nutrient deficiency and for the prevention of deficiency in certain 'at risk' groups of the population. These are the only prescribable indications for vitamins and minerals on the NHS.

But what is a balanced diet? And how many people consume such a diet? The fact that deficiency diseases such as scurvy have been largely eradicated in Britain seems to suggest that the diet is adequate. However, it has been suggested that marginal deficiency is a problem which often goes unrecognized, particularly in some groups of the population, e.g. the elderly, individuals on low incomes and smokers.

Assessment of deficiency

Deficiency may be assessed by measurement of various indices (e.g. enzyme activities, blood levels and urinary excretion) but these do not always accurately reflect tissue stores. In cases of severe deficiency there may be clear clinical signs and symptoms, but marginal or subclinical deficiency is more difficult to assess as signs and symptoms are often vague and non-specific.

Groups at risk of deficiency

These include:

- people in a particular demographic category, e.g. infants and children, adolescents, women during pregnancy and lactation and throughout the reproductive period, the elderly and ethnic minorities;
- people whose nutritional status may be compromised by lifestyle (enforced or voluntary), e.g. smokers, alcoholics, drug addicts, slimmers, strict vegetarians (i.e. vegans), food faddists, individuals on low incomes and athletes; however, people with diabetes mellitus do not normally need supplements;
- people whose nutritional status may be compromised by surgery and/or disease, e.g. malabsorption syndromes, hepato-biliary disorders, severe burns and wounds and inborn errors of metabolism; and
- people whose nutritional status may be compromised by long-term drug administration (e.g. anticonvulsants may increase the requirement for vitamin D).

Clearly, these groups encompass nearly every individual except some adult males. However, deficiency is only likely if the individual has two or three risk factors. Such individuals may benefit from supplements.

Problems with supplements

The arguments against the use of supplements are several:

- firstly they can induce complacency and encourage the consumption of a poor diet;
- secondly many people who use supplements are extremely health conscious and already eat a good diet and so are the least likely to need supplementation;
- thirdly they are unnecessary because deficiency disorders (e.g. scurvy) have largely disappeared in the UK; and
- fourthly, cost.

Other concerns include the potential to mislead consumers (discussed earlier) and the possible presence of contaminants.

More important is the fact that many supplements contain nutrients which can cause toxicity when taken in excessive amounts (see Table 2.4). A Ministry of Agriculture, Fisheries and Food/Department of Health Working Group recommended limits for the maximum daily doses of micronutrients in dietary supplements. These proposed limits are also shown in Table 2.4.

Table 2.4 Toxic doses of nutrients

	RNI[1]	Toxic dose/d	Maximum levels[2]
Vitamins			
Vitamin A	700 μg	6 mg	600 μg
(as retinol)	(2310 units)	(19 800 units)	(1980 units)
Niacin	17 mg		50 mg
Nicotinic acid		3–9 g	
Nicotinamide (s/r[3])		500 mg	
Vitamin B_6	1.4 mg	50 mg	10 mg
Vitamin C	40 mg	6 g	600 mg
Vitamin D	–	500 μg	5 μg
		(20 000 units)	(200 units)
Minerals			
Chromium	–	1–2 g	100 mg
Cobalt	–	300 mg	30 mg
Copper	1.2 mg	50 μg/kg	3 mg
Fluorine	–	10 mg	1 mg
Germanium	–	20 mg	
Iron	8.7 mg	40 mg	4 mg
Iodine	140 μg	1000 μg	1000 μg
Molybdenum	–	10–15 mg	1 mg
Nickel	–	250 mg	
Selenium	75 μg	1 mg	1000 μg
Zinc	9.5 mg	20 mg	2 mg

1. RNI for men aged 19–50 years
2. Maximum daily doses of vitamins and minerals in dietary supplements recommended by MAFF (1991)
3. Sustained release

There is also a danger in giving undue emphasis to individual nutrients that just happen to be fashionable at a given time. The 1930s and 1940s were the era of iron and iodine; vitamin C and zinc both became popular in the 1970s, calcium and selenium in the 1980s and betacarotene in the 1990s.

An exclusive concern with individual nutrients is potentially dangerous. It can result in pronounced changes in human exposure to such nutrients, creating a risk of imbalances. Nutritional balance can be disturbed not only by deficiencies but also by excessive intake of certain nutrients which, although not toxic in and of themselves, can adversely affect the bioavailability and function of others. Vitamins and minerals do not work in isolation; they behave as a highly interactive network. In addition, it is rare to be deficient in one nutrient; several are usually involved.

Patient/client counselling

The following questions may be used by health professionals before making any recommendations about supplement use:

1. *Who is the supplement for?* The individual buying the product may not be the consumer; requirements for vitamins and minerals vary according to age and sex.

2. *Why do you think you need a supplement?* The individual may have misconceptions about the need for and benefits of supplements that should be addressed.

3. *What are your symptoms (if any) and how long have you had them?* The individual could have a serious underlying disorder that should be referred for appropriate diagnosis and treatment.

4. *What do you eat?* A simple dietary assessment should be undertaken to give some indication whether vitamin and mineral deficiency is likely.

5. *Is your diet restricted in any way?* Slimming, vegetarianism or religious conviction could increase the risk of nutritional deficiency.

6. Do you take any prescription or over-the-counter medicines? This information can be used to assess possible drug-nutrient interactions.

7. *Do you take other supplements? If so, which ones?* This information can be used to assess potential overdosage of supplements which could be toxic.

8. *Do you suffer from any chronic illness e.g. Crohn's disease, cancer?* Nutrient requirements in patients with chronic disease may be greater than in healthy individuals. Some supplements are contra-indicated in certain diseases.

9. *Are you pregnant or breast-feeding?* Nutrient requirements may be increased. Some supplements are contra-indicated during pregnancy and lactation.

10. *Do you take part in sports or other regular physical activity?*

11. *Do you smoke?* Requirements for some vitamins (e.g. vitamin C) may be increased.

12. *How much alcohol do you drink?* Excessive alcohol consumption may lead to deficiency of the B vitamins.

Guidelines for supplement use

The following guidelines may be useful in making recommendations:

- compare labels with dietary standards (usually RDAs),
- in the absence of an indication for a specific nutrient, a balanced multivitamin/mineral product is normally preferable to one which contains one or two specific nutrients,
- use a product that provides approximately 100% of the RDA for as wide a range of vitamins and minerals as possible,

- avoid preparations containing unrecognized nutrients or nutrients in minute amounts (this increases the cost, but not the value), and
- avoid preparations which claim to be natural, organic, or high-potency (this increases the cost and, in the case of high-potency products, the risk of toxicity).

Supplements should not be used as a substitute for healthy eating for prolonged periods of time. They do not convert a poor diet into a good one.

Role of the health professional

When asked about supplements, health professionals should emphasize the importance of consuming a diet based on healthy eating guidelines. This is a diet rich in starchy, fibrous carbohydrates, including fruit and vegetables, and low in fat, sugar and salt.

Health professionals should be aware of dietary standards and good food sources for nutrients. They should be able to assess an individual's risk of nutrient deficiency, and need for further referral, by asking questions to detect cultural, physical, environmental and social conditions which may predispose to inadequate intakes.

There is a need to be aware of the potential for adverse effects with supplements. Thus, when a client or patient presents with any symptoms, questions should be asked about the use of dietary supplements. Individuals will not always volunteer this information without prompting because they believe that supplements are 'natural' and therefore safe.

Health professionals should make their clients aware of the existence of badly worded claims and advertisements, and of the dangers of supplement misuse.

Pharmacists have a particular responsibility, simply because they sell these products. When supplying any supplement with perceived health benefits, pharmacists must be careful to avoid giving their professional authority to a product which may lack any health or therapeutic benefit or has risks associated with its use. In accordance with the Code of Ethics of the Royal Pharmaceutical Society of Great Britain, this may involve not stocking or selling the product. Pharmacists must not give the impression that any dietary supplement is efficacious when there is no evidence for such efficacy.

However, providing a product is not harmful for a particular individual, the freedom to use it should be respected. What is important is that consumers are able to make informed and intelligent choices about the products they buy.

References and further reading

Anonymous (1990) Natural alternatives. *Which? Way to Health* June, 80–1.
Anonymous (1992) Multivitamin tablets. Who needs them? *Which? Way to Health* August, 123–5.
Anonymous (1993) Dietary supplements: rationale for regulation. *Nutr Rev* **51**, 310–2.
Anonymous (1994) Evening primrose oil – is it for you? *Which? Way to health* April, 66–7.
Bender A.E. (1985) *Health or Hoax.* Elvendon Press, Reading.
Bender D.A. (1992) *Nutritional biochemistry of the vitamins.* Cambridge University Press, Cambridge.

Benn Publications (1994) *The OTC Healthcare Report.* Benn Publications Ltd, Tonbridge, Kent.
Council on Scientific Affairs (1987) Vitamin preparations as dietary supplements and as therapeutic agents. *J Am Med Ass* **257**, 1929–36.
DHSS (1969) *Recommended intakes of nutrients for the United Kingdom. Report on Public Health and Medical Subjects No. 120.* HMSO, London.
DHSS (1979) *Recommended daily amounts of food energy and nutrients for groups of people in the United Kingdom. Report on Health and Social Subjects No. 15.* HMSO, London.
DoH (1991) *Dietary Reference Values for food energy and nutrients for the United Kingdom. Report on Health and Social Subjects No. 41.* HMSO, London.
Evans D.H. & Lacey J.H. (1986) Toxicity of vitamins: complications of a health movement. *Br Med J* **292**, 509–10.
Gaby S.K., Bendich A., Singh V.N. & Machlin L.J. (eds) (1991) *Vitamin Intake and Health.* Marcel Dekker, New York.
Machlin, L.J. (ed.) (1990): *Handbook of Vitamins*, 2nd edn, Marcel Dekker, New York.
MAFF/DoH (1991) *Dietary Supplements and Health Foods. Report of a working group.* MAFF Publications, London.
National Research Council, Food and Nutrition Board, Commission on Life Sciences (1989) *Recommended dietary allowances*, 10th edn, National Academy Press, Washington DC.
Nelson M.V. (1988) Promotion and Selling of Unnecessary Food Supplements: Quackery or Ethical Pharmacy Practice? *American Pharmacy* **NS28**, 34–6.
Ovesen L. (1984) Vitamin Therapy in the Absence of Obvious Deficiency. What is the Evidence? *Drugs* **27**, 148–70.
Roe D, (1994) *Handbook on Drug and Nutrient Interactions.* 5th edn, American Dietetic Association, Chicago.
Shils M., Olson J. & Shike M. (eds) *Modern Nutrition in Health and Disease* 8th edn, Lea & Febiger, Philadelphia.
Truswell S. (1990) Who should take vitamin supplements? *Br Med J* **301**, 135–6.
World Health Organisation Regional Office for Europe (1993) *Use and Regulation of Vitamin and Mineral Supplements. A Study with Policy Recommendations.* Styx Publications, Groningen, The Netherlands.

Chapter 3
Antioxidants

Description

Various antioxidant systems have evolved to offer protection against free radicals and prevent damage to vital biological structures such as lipid membranes, proteins and DNA. Antioxidant capacity is a concept which is used to describe the overall ability of tissues to inhibit free-radical-mediated processes (Jackson 1994). It is dependent on the concentrations of individual antioxidants and activity of protective enzymes.

The commonest and most important antioxidant defences are shown in Table 3.1.

Table 3.1 Anti-oxidant defences

Intracellular antioxidants
 Enzymes
  catalase
  glutathione peroxidase
  superoxide dismutase

Extracellular antioxidants
 Vitamin C
 Sulphydryl groups

Membrane antioxidants
 Carotenoids
 Ubiquinone
 Vitamin E

Substances essential for synthesis of antioxidant enzymes
 Copper
 Manganese
 Selenium
 Zinc

The antioxidant vitamins can be divided into those that are water-soluble and exist in aqueous solution – primarily vitamin C – and those that are fat-soluble and exist in membranes or lipoproteins – vitamin E and betacarotene. Lipid membranes are particularly vulnerable to oxidative breakdown by free radicals. Vitamin E protects cell membranes from destruction by undergoing preferential oxidation and destruction. Some quinones, such as ubiquinone (coenzyme Q) also appear to have antioxidant properties. All these substances can act as free radical scavengers and can react directly with free radicals.

Some trace elements act as essential components of antioxidant enzymes;

copper, magnesium or zinc for superoxide dismutase and selenium for glutathione peroxidase.

Action

Antioxidants are believed to protect against certain diseases by preventing the deleterious effects of free-radical-mediated processes in cell membranes and by reducing the susceptibility of tissues to oxidative stress.

Free radicals

Each orbital surrounding the nucleus of an atom is occupied by a pair of electrons. If an orbital in the outer shell of a molecule loses an electron, the molecule becomes a free radical. As a result of the unpaired electron, the molecule becomes unstable and, therefore, highly reactive. The free radical may then react with any other nearby molecule also converting that molecule to a free radical which can then initiate another reaction. Some free radicals are capable of severely damaging cells.

Theoretically, a single free radical can ultimately cause an endless number of reactions. This chain reaction is terminated either by the free radical's reaction with another free radical, resulting in the formation of a covalently bound molecule, or by the free radical's reaction with an antioxidant, an antioxidant enzyme, or both. Fortunately, many enzyme systems have evolved to provide protection from free radical production.

Because antioxidant defences are not completely efficient, increased free radical formation in the body is likely to increase damage. The term 'oxidative stress' is often used to refer to this effect. If mild oxidative stress occurs, tissues often respond by increasing their antioxidant defences. However, severe oxidative stress can cause cell injury and cell death.

There is growing evidence that free radical damage is involved in the development of many diseases, such as atherosclerosis (Witztum 1994), cancer (Cerutti 1994), Parkinson's disease and other neurodegenerative disorders (Jenner 1994), inflammatory bowel disease (Grisham 1994) and lung disease (Cross *et al.* 1994).

Uses

Epidemiological evidence is emerging that low plasma levels of antioxidant nutrients and low dietary intakes are related to an increased risk of diseases such as coronary heart disease and cancer. There is also increasing evidence that these diseases can be prevented or delayed to some extent by dietary changes, in particular by increased consumption of fruits and vegetables. Several substances in fruit and vegetables (e.g. betacarotene, vitamin C and vitamin E) may act to diminish oxidative damage *in vivo* and, because our endogenous antioxidant defences are not completely effective, dietary antioxidants may be important in diminishing the cumulative effects of oxidative damage in the human body.

A question of particular current interest is whether supplementation of adequately nourished subjects with antioxidant nutrients will reduce the incidence of such diseases. The few intervention trials of antioxidants reported so far have shown little evidence for the value of supplements. However, further large trials are now in progress.

Cardiovascular disease

Experimental studies suggest an inverse association between CHD mortality and vitamin C, vitamin E and betacarotene and argue strongly in favour of a protective role of antioxidants in the development of atherosclerosis.

In a cross-cultural study of middle-aged men representing 16 European populations (Gey *et al.* 1991) differences in mortality from ischaemic heart disease were primarily attributable to plasma levels of vitamin E. Twelve of the 16 populations had similar blood cholesterol and blood pressure but differed greatly in tocopherol levels and heart disease death rates. For vitamin E, mean plasma levels lower than 25 micromoles/litre were associated with a high risk of coronary heart disease, whereas plasma levels above this value were associated with a lower risk of disease. In the case of vitamin C, mean plasma levels less than 22.7 micromoles/L were found in those regions that had a moderate to high risk of disease, whereas plasma levels in excess of this level tended to be found in those areas at low risk.

In a large case control study in Scotland (Riemersma *et al.* 1991), 6000 men aged 35–54 were studied for a possible association between anti-oxidant status and risk of angina pectoris. Highly significant correlations between low plasma concentrations of betacarotene, vitamin C and vitamin E and risk of angina were found.

The Health Professionals Study (Rimm *et al.* 1993), a large prospective investigation, which looked at 39 910 US male health professionals aged 40–75 years, showed that men who took more than 100 units of vitamin E daily for over two years had a 37% reduction in risk of heart disease. The Nurses' Health Study (Stampfer *et al.* 1993), in which 87 245 female nurses aged 34–59 years took part, showed that women who took more than 200 units of vitamin E daily for more than two years had a 41% reduction in risk of coronary heart disease.

The only intervention trial published so far (in the form of an abstract), a study of 333 male physicians aged between 40 and 84 years with angina pectoris and/or coronary revascularisation, showed that 50 mg of beta-carotene on alternate days resulted in a 44% reduction in major coronary events (Gaziano *et al.* 1990).

Cancer

There is now good evidence linking high intake of fruit and vegetables with lower incidence of certain cancers, and it is presumed that the protective nutrients are some or all of the antioxidant nutrients.

In a study of 25 802 volunteers in Washington County, Maryland (Comstock *et al.* 1991) prediagnostic blood samples from 436 cancer cases at nine cancer sites were compared with 765 matched control cases. Serum betacarotene levels showed a strong protective association with lung cancer, suggestive protective associations with melanoma and bladder cancer, and a suggestive but nonprotective association with rectal cancer. Serum vitamin E levels showed a protective association with lung cancer, but none of the other cancer sites studied showed impressive associations. Low levels of serum lycopene (a carotenoid occurring in ripe fruits) were strongly associated with pancreatic cancer and less strongly associated with cancer of the bladder and rectum.

The Basel study from Switzerland (Stahelin *et al.* 1991) demonstrated that patients who had died from all cancers, including bronchus cancer and stomach cancer, had statistically lower mean carotene levels compared with a matched group of healthy survivors.

In a Finnish study (Knekt *et al*. 1991), individuals with low serum levels of vitamin E had about a 1.5-fold risk of cancer compared with those with a higher serum level of vitamin E. The strength of the association between serum vitamin E level and cancer risk varied for different cancer sites and was strongest for some gastro-intestinal cancers and for the combined group of cancers unrelated to smoking.

An intervention trial in Linxian, China (Blot *et al*. 1993) has provided much needed clinical data on the effects of specific vitamin-mineral supplementation on cancer incidence and disease-specific mortality. Linxian County has one of the world's highest rates of oesophageal and gastric cancers. Combined daily doses of 15 mg betacarotene, 30 mg vitamin E and 50 µg selenium taken over five years were associated with a 13% reduction in deaths from cancer and an overall reduction in mortality of 9%.

These results, although impressive and worthy of further investigation, might have been achieved because the population studied had low intakes and were deficient in the nutrients investigated. A similar study is required in a well-nourished population.

Not all studies have shown positive results. The ATBC study in Finland (The Alpha-Tocopherol, Beta Carotene Cancer Prevention Study Group 1994) found no reduction in the incidence of lung cancer among male smokers after five to eight years of dietary supplementation with vitamin E or betacarotene; a higher incidence of lung cancer was observed in the group receiving betacarotene.

However, these results should be considered in the context of the population studied – the subjects had smoked an average of 20 cigarettes a day for 36 years. Most studies with antioxidants suggest that their protective properties are associated with the early stages of cancer and it is likely that this intervention took place too late in the carcinogenic process. In addition, the study could have employed too low a dosage (50 mg vitamin E and/or 20 mg betacarotene were used) or was of too short a duration. Nevertheless, this increased incidence of lung cancer in the group receiving betacarotene cannot be ignored.

In the Nurses' Health Study (Hunter *et al*. 1993), large intakes of vitamin C or E did not protect women from breast cancer. In contrast, there was a significant inverse association of vitamin A intake with risk of this disease. The authors concluded, however, that vitamin A supplements are unlikely to influence the risk of breast cancer among women whose dietary intake of this vitamin is already adequate.

In the Polyp Prevention Study (Greenberg *et al*. 1994) there was no evidence that supplements of betacarotene, or vitamins C and E reduced the incidence of colorectal adenomas.

Cataract

Incidence of cataract is now also being investigated for links with anti-oxidants. Low vitamin C intakes have been associated with increased risk of cataract (Jaques & Chylack 1991). Increased levels of supplementary vitamins C and E correlated with a 50% reduction in the risk of cataracts

(Robertson *et al.* 1991). The Nurses' Health Study (Hankinson *et al.* 1992) found that dietary carotenoids, although not necessarily betacarotene, and long term vitamin C supplementation may reduce the risk of cataracts.

Conclusion

Biochemical evidence suggests that oxidative stress caused by accumulation of free radicals is involved in the pathogenesis of several diseases. Appropriate levels of antioxidant nutrients might therefore be expected to delay or prevent these diseases. Several epidemiological studies have found lower serum levels of antioxidant nutrients in patients with cardiovascular disease, cancer and cataract but there is, as yet, little evidence that supplements of antioxidant nutrients prevent disease. Further intervention trials are needed. In the meantime, the best advice to give is to eat plenty of fruit and vegetables (five or more servings a day).

References

The Alpha-Tocopherol, Beta Carotene Cancer Prevention Study Group (1994) The effect of vitamin E and beta carotene on the incidence of lung cancer in male smokers. *New Engl J Med* **330**, 1029–35.

Blot W.J., Li J.Y., Taylor P.R. *et al.* (1993) Nutrition intervention trials in Linxian, China: supplementation with specific vitamin/mineral combinations, cancer incidence, and disease-specific mortality in the general population. *J Natl Cancer Inst* **85**, 1483–92.

Cerutti P.A. (1994) Oxy-radicals and cancer. *Lancet* **344**, 862–3.

Comstock G.W., Helzlsouer K.J. & Bush T. (1991) Prediagnostic serum levels of carotenoids and vitamin E as related to subsequent cancer in Washington County, Maryland. *Am J Clin Nutr* **53**, 260S–4S.

Cross C.E., van der Vliet A., O'Neill C.A. & Eiserich J.P. (1994) Reactive oxygen species and the lung. *Lancet* **344**, 930–3.

Gaziano J.M., Manson J.E., Ridker P.M., Buring J.E. & Hennekens C.H. (1990) Beta carotene therapy for chronic stable angina. *Circulation* **82**, Suppl III, 201, Abstr. 0796.

Gey K.F., Puska P., Jordan P. & Moser UK (1991) Inverse correlation between plasma vitamin E and mortality from ischaemic heart disease in cross-cultural epidemiology. *Am J Clin Nutr* **53**, 326S–34S.

Greenberg E.R., Baron J.A., Tosteson T.D. *et al.* (1994) A clinical trial of antioxidant vitamins to prevent colorectal adenoma. *New Engl J Med* **331**, 141–7.

Grisham M.B. (1994) Oxidants and free radicals in inflammatory bowel disease. *Lancet* **344**, 859–61.

Hankinson S.E., Stampfer M.J., Seddon J.M., Colditz G.A., Rosner B., Speizer F.E. & Willett W.C. (1992) Nutrient intake and cataract extraction in women: a prospective study. *Br Med J* **305**, 335–9.

Hunter D.J., Manson J.E., Colditz G.A., Stampfer M.J., Rosner B., Hennekens C.H., Speizer F.E. & Willett W. (1993) A prospective study of vitamins C, E and A and the risk of breast cancer. *New Engl J Med* **329**, 234–40.

Jackson M.J. (1994) Can dietary micronutrients influence tissue antioxidant capacity? *Proc Nutr Soc* **53**, 53–7.

Jacques P.F. & Chylack L.T. (1991) Epidemiologic evidence of a role for the antioxidant vitamins and carotenoids in cancer prevention. *Am J Clin Nutr* **53**, 352S–5S.

Jenner P. (1994) Oxidative damage in neurodegenerative disease. *Lancet* **344**, 796–8.

Knekt P., Aromaa A., Maatela J., Aaran R-K., Nikkari T., Hakama M., Hakulinen T.,

Peto R. & Teppo L. (1991) Vitamin E and cancer prevention. *Am J Clin Nutr* **53**, 283S–6S.

Riemersma R.A., Wood D.A., MacIntyre C.C.A., Elton R.A., Gey K.F. & Oliver M.F. (1991) Risk of angina pectoris and plasma concentrations of vitamins A, C and E and carotene. *Lancet* **337**, 1–5.

Rimm E.B., Stampfer M.J., Ascherio A., Giovannucci E., Colditz G. & Willett W. (1993) Vitamin E consumption and the risk of coronary heart disease in men. *New Engl J Med* **328**, 1450–6.

Robertson J. McD., Donner A.P. & Trevithick J.R. (1991) A possible role for vitamins C and E in cataract prevention. *Am J Clin Nutr* **53**, 346S–51S.

Stahelin H.B., Gey K.F., Eichholzer M. & Ludin E. (1991) β-carotene and cancer prevention: the Basel study. *Am J Clin Nutr* **53**, 265S–9S.

Stampfer M.J., Hennekens C.H., Manson J.E., Colditz G.A., Rosner B. & Willett W. (1993) Vitamin E consumption and the risk of coronary heart disease in women. *New Engl J Med* **328**, 1444–9.

Witzum J.L. (1994) The oxidation hypothesis of atherosclerosis. *Lancet* **344**, 793–5.

Chapter 4
Bioflavonoids

Description and nomenclature
Bioflavonoids are sometimes known as vitamin P substances. They do not belong to an officially recognized group of vitamins.

Constituents
Bioflavonoids are a group of polyphenolic antioxidants which often occur as glycosides. They include the anthocyanins, catechins, flavanones, flavones (e.g. apigenin and luteolin) and flavonols (e.g. kaempferol, quercetin and myricetin).

Human requirements
No proof of a dietary need exists.

Intakes
In the UK the average adult diet provides 1 g daily.

Dietary sources
Bioflavonoids are found in the white segment or ring of fruit (especially citrus fruit) and vegetables, and also in tea and wine.

Action
Bioflavonoids appear to display several effects (Hertog et al. 1993). They:

- act as scavengers of free radicals (including superoxide anions, singlet oxygen, and lipid peroxy radicals);
- sequester metal ions;
- inhibit in vitro oxidation of low density lipoproteins (LDL);
- inhibit cyclo-oxygenase, leading to lower platelet aggregation, decreased thrombotic tendency and reduced anti-inflammatory activity;
- inhibit histamine release; and
- improve capillary function by reducing fragility of capillary walls and thus preventing abnormal leakage.

Uses

Cardiovascular disease
Bioflavonoids may help to reduce the risk of heart disease (possibly by helping to dilate the coronary arteries and by preventing atherosclerosis). A study from the Netherlands (Hertog et al. 1993) demonstrated a reduced risk of coronary heart disease and a reduced incidence of myocardial infarction in men associated with increased ingestion of dietary flavonoids.

The major dietary source of flavonoids in this study was tea, and other antioxidant polyphenols present in tea could have influenced the result. Other studies to confirm these observations are needed in other populations and in groups where the majority of flavonoid intake is provided by other dietary constituents apart from tea.

Cancer

Activity of flavonoids against malignant cells has also been demonstrated *in vitro* (Havsteen 1983; Tripathi & Rastogi 1981) and there is much current interest in the potential use of bioflavonoids in the prevention and treatment of cancer.

Cataract

There may be a role for flavonoids in preventing diabetes-related cataract formation. In diabetes mellitus, excess sorbitol or dulcitol is produced by the conversion of glucose by aldose reductase. The dulcitol cannot be further metabolized and therefore forms a hard crystalline layer in the lens, the cataract. Flavonoids are potent inhibitors of the enzyme (Wagner 1977), but further studies are required before flavonoids could be recommended for cataract prevention.

Miscellaneous

Experimental studies have demonstrated that some flavonoids prevent ulcer formation (Farkas *et al*. 1981), and that they may be useful in treating ulcers.

Flavonoids have been investigated for potential anti-viral activity. *In vitro* tests have shown some activity against rhinovirus (responsible for 50% of common colds) but little activity against Herpes Simplex and influenza virus (Tshuiya *et al*. 1985).

Many claims have been made for the usefulness of bioflavonoids in a range of disorders, including haemorrhoids, allergy, asthma, menopausal symptoms and the prevention of habitual abortion, but scientific studies are required to investigate these claims.

Pregnancy and breast-feeding

No problems reported.

Adverse effects

None reported.

Dose

• Not established; dietary supplements provide 250–500 µg in a single dose.

References

Farkas L., Gabor M., Kallay F. & Wagner H. (1981) Flavonoids and bioflavonoids. *Proc Int Bioflav Sym*, Munich. Elsevier, Amsterdam.

Havsteen B. (1983) Flavonoids. A class of natural products of high pharmacological potency. *Biochem Pharmacol* **32**, 1141.

Hertog M.G.L, Feskens E.J.M., Hollman P.C.H., Katan M.B. & Kromhout D. (1993) Dietary antioxidant flavonoids and risk of coronary heart disease: the Zutphen elderly study. *Lancet* **342**, 1007–11.

Tripathi V.D. & Rastogi R.P. (1981) Flavonoids in biology and medicine. *J Sci Ind Res* **40**, 116.

Tshuiya Y., Shimuzu M., Hiyama Y., Itoh K., Hashimoto Y., Nagayama M., Horie T. & Morita M. (1985) Antiviral activity of naturally occurring flavonoids in vitro. *Chem Pharm Bull* **33**, 3881.

Wagner H. (1977) Phenolic compounds of pharmaceutical interest. In *Recent Advances in Phytochemistry, Volume 12, Biochemistry of Plant Phenolics*, 589.

Chapter 5
Biotin

Description
Biotin is a water-soluble vitamin and a member of the vitamin B complex.

Nomenclature
Biotin was formerly known as vitamin H or coenzyme R.

Human requirements
In the UK no Reference Nutrient Intake or Estimated Average Requirement has been set. A safe and adequate intake is 10–200 µg daily.

Intakes
In the UK, the average adult diet provides 33 µg daily. Biotin is also produced by colonic bacteria, but the effect of this on biotin requirements is not known.

Action
Biotin functions as an integral part of the enzymes that transport carboxyl units and fix carbon dioxide. Biotin enzymes are important in carbohydrate and lipid metabolism and are involved in gluconeogenesis, fatty acid synthesis, propionate metabolism and catabolism of amino acids.

Dietary sources
Biotin is ubiquitous in the diet. The richest sources of biotin are liver, kidney, eggs, soya beans and peanuts. Meat, wholegrain cereals, wholemeal bread, milk and cheese are also good sources. Green vegetables contain very little biotin.

Metabolism

Absorption
Biotin is absorbed rapidly from the gastro-intestinal tract by facilitated transport (at low concentrations) and by passive diffusion (at high concentrations). Absorption is greater in the jejunum than the ileum and minimal in the colon.

Distribution
Biotin is bound to plasma proteins.

Elimination
Excess biotin is excreted largely unchanged in the urine. It also appears in breast milk.

Deficiency

Biotin deficiency is a risk only in those patients on prolonged parenteral nutrition (who will automatically be given multi-vitamin supplements). Deficiency has been induced by the addition of large amounts of raw egg white, which contains the biotin-binding protein, avidin, to a diet low in biotin (Baugh *et al.* 1968).

Symptoms of biotin deficiency include:

- anorexia,
- nausea,
- vomiting,
- dry scaly dermatitis,
- glossitis,
- loss of taste,
- somnolence,
- panic, and
- an increase in serum cholesterol and bile pigments.

Uses

Biotin has been claimed to be of value in the treatment of brittle finger nails, acne, seborrhoeic dermatitis, hair fragility and alopecia, but such claims need further confirmation by controlled clinical trials.

Biotin deficiency has been associated with sudden infant death syndrome (SIDS). In one study, the median biotin levels in the livers of infants who died from SIDS were significantly lower than those of infants who died from explicable causes (Heard *et al.* 1983). However, evidence that biotin deficiency is an important contributory factor in SIDS is circumstantial and unequivocal proof is lacking. There is no requirement for biotin supplements in newborn or young infants. Supplements should NOT be sold to parents for this purpose.

Pregnancy and breast-feeding

No problems reported.

Adverse effects

None reported.

Interactions

Drugs

Anticonvulsants (carbamazepine, phenobarbitone, phenytoin and primidone): requirements for biotin may be increased.

Dose

None established; dietary supplements provide 100–300 µg in a daily dose.

References

Baugh C.M., Malone J.W., Butterworth, C.E. Jr (1968) Human biotin deficiency. A case history of biotin deficiency induced by raw egg consumption in a cirrhotic patient. *Am J Clin Nutr*, **21**: 173–82.

Heard G.S., Hood R.L. & Johnson A.R. (1983). Hepatic biotin and sudden infant death syndrome. *Med J Aust* **2**: 305–6.

Chapter 6
Bonemeal

Description

Bone meal is ground animal bone.

Constituents

The main constituent is calcium hydroxyapatite which provides calcium and phosphorus. Bonemeal also contains traces of magnesium.

Uses

Bonemeal is used as a source of calcium.

Precautions/contra-indications

Bone meal may be contaminated with cadmium, lead and/or mercury (Robert 1983). Supplements should be avoided.

Pregnancy and breast-feeding

Avoid (contaminants – see Precautions).

Adverse effects

None (except contaminants – see Precautions).

Interactions

See calcium (Section 9).

Dose

Dietary supplements provide 250–500 mg calcium per dose.

References

Robert S.H.J. (1983) Potential toxicity due to dolomite and bonemeal. *South Med J* **76**, 556–9.

Chapter 7
Boron

Description
Boron is an ultratrace mineral.

Human requirements
Evidence is accumulating that boron is an essential nutrient for humans, but requirements have not so far been defined.

Intakes
Most UK diets appear to provide about 2 mg daily.

Action
Boron appears to be important in calcium metabolism and can affect the composition, structure and strength of bone. It influences the metabolism of calcium, copper, magnesium, phosphorus, potassium and vitamin D.

In addition, boron affects the activity of certain enzymes. It also affects brain function; boron deprivation appears to depress mental alertness (Nielsen 1993).

Dietary sources
Foods of plant origin, especially fruits, vegetables and nuts, are rich sources of boron, but there is little in meat, fish and poultry. Beer, wine and cider contain significant amounts.

Metabolism

Absorption
Dietary boron is rapidly absorbed. The mechanism of absorption from the gastro-intestinal tract has not been elucidated.

Distribution
Boron is distributed throughout the body tissues; the highest concentrations are found in the bone, spleen and thyroid.

Elimination
Boron is excreted mainly in the urine.

Deficiency
No precise signs and symptoms of boron deficiency have been defined.

Uses

Boron may have beneficial effects on calcium metabolism in post-menopausal women by preventing calcium loss and bone demineralization. In a study of 12 post-menopausal women (Nielsen *et al.* 1987) boron supplementation (3 mg daily) reduced urinary excretions of calcium and magnesium and elevated serum concentrations of oestradiol and ionized calcium.

A further study (Nielsen *et al.* 1990) has provided evidence that boron can both enhance and mimic some effects of oestrogen ingestion in post-menopausal women. In women receiving oestrogen therapy an increase in boron intake increased serum oestradiol concentrations to higher levels than when boron intake was low. These effects did not occur in men, or in women not receiving oestrogen therapy. These findings support the contention that, if oestrogen is beneficial to calcium metabolism, then boron might also be beneficial.

Boron has been claimed to relieve the symptoms of arthritis, but scientific studies are required.

Pregnancy and breast-feeding

No problems reported, but caution because of possible changes in oestrogen metabolism.

Adverse effects

Boron is relatively non-toxic when administered orally at doses contained in food supplements. High oral doses (> 100 mg daily) are associated with:

- disturbances in appetite and digestion,
- nausea,
- vomiting,
- diarrhoea,
- dermatitis and
- lethargy.

Toxicity has occurred, especially in children, from the application of boron-containing dusting powders and lotions (in the form of borax or boric acid) to areas of broken skin and mucous membranes. Such preparations are no longer recommended.

Interactions

Nutrients

Riboflavin: large doses increase excretion of riboflavin.

Dose

Not established; dietary supplements provide on average 3 mg per daily dose.

References

Nielsen F.H., Hunt C.D., Mullen L.M. & Hunt J.R. (1987) Effect of dietary boron on mineral, estrogen and testosterone metabolism in postmenopausal women. *FASEB J* 1: 394–7.
Nielsen F.H., Mullen L.M. & Gallagher S.K. (1990) Effect of boron depletion and

repletion on blood indicators of calcium status in humans fed a magnesium-low diet. *J Trace Elem Exp Med* **3**: 45–54.

Nielsen F.H. (1993) In: *Modern Nutrition in Health and Disease* (eds M. Shils, J. Olson & M. Shike), 8th edn, p 274. Len & Febiger, Philadelphia.

Chapter 8
Brewer's Yeast

Nomenclature

Saccharomyces cerevisiae.

Constituents

Average Nutrient Composition of Dried Brewer's Yeast

Nutrient	Per teaspoon (8 g)	% RNI[1] (approx)
Vitamin A	Trace	—
Thiamin	1.2 mg	133 mg
Riboflavin	0.4 mg	33 mg
Niacin	2.0 mg	14 mg
Vitamin B_6	0.2 mg	16 mg
Folic acid	320 µg	160 µg
Pantothenic acid	0.9 mg	—
Biotin	16 µg	—
Vitamin C	Trace	—
Calcium	6 mg	0.9 mg
Magnesium	18 mg	6 mg
Potassium	160 mg	4.5 mg
Phosphorus	103 mg	19 mg
Iron	1.6 mg	13 mg
Zinc	0.6 mg	7 mg
Copper	0.4 mg	33 mg

1. Reference Nutrient Intake for men aged 19–50 years
Note: Brewer's yeast tablets contain approximately 300 mg brewer's yeast per tablet; extra B vitamins are often added. Brewer's yeast is also claimed to contain significant quantities of chromium and selenium.

Uses

Brewer's yeast is a useful source of B vitamins and several minerals (see Constituents).

Brewer's yeast has been used to treat diarrhoea due to *Clostridium difficile* (Schellenberg *et al.* 1994). Because brewer's yeast contains chromium it has been claimed to help in the control of blood glucose levels. It is also claimed to prevent hypercholesterolaemia. However, there is insufficient evidence for these claims.

Precautions/contra-indications

Brewer's yeast should be avoided by patients taking monoamine oxidase inhibitors (see Interactions). It is also best avoided by patients with gout; this is because of high concentrations of nucleic acids which may lead to purine formation.

Pregnancy and breast-feeding
No problems reported.

Adverse effects
None reported except flatulence.

Interactions
Monoamine oxidase inhibitors: may provoke hypertensive crisis.

Dose
Not established.

References
Schellenberg D., Bonington A., Champion C.M., Lancaster R., Webb S. & Main J. (1994) Treatment of Clostridium difficile diarrhoea with brewer's yeast. *Lancet* **343**: 171.

Chapter 9
Calcium

Description
Calcium is an essential mineral.

Human requirements
Dietary Reference Values (mg/d)

Age	RNI	EAR	LRNI
0–12 months	525	400	240
1–3 years	350	275	200
4–6 years	450	350	275
7–10 years	550	425	325
Male			
11–18 years	1000	750	450
19–50+ years	700	525	400
Female			
11–18 years	800	625	480
19–50+	700	525	400
Pregnancy	800	625	480
Lactation	1350	—	—

Note: The National Osteoporosis Society has produced separate guidelines for recommended daily calcium intake as follows: 7–12 years, 800 mg; 13–19 years, 1000 mg; men 20–45 years, 1000 mg; men > 45 years, 1500 mg; women 20–45 years, 1000 mg; women > 45 years, 1500 mg; women > 45 years (using Hormone Replacement Therapy), 1000 mg; pregnant and breast-feeding women, 1200 mg; pregnant and breast-feeding teenagers, 1500 mg.
Reproduced and adapted with the permission of the Controller of Her Majesty's Stationery Office.

Intakes
In the UK the average diet provides: for men, 961 mg daily; women, 764 mg daily.

Action
Calcium has a structural role in bones and teeth. It is also essential for cellular structure, blood clotting, muscle contraction, nerve transmission, enzyme activation and hormone function.

Dietary sources

Food portion	Calcium content (mg)
Cereal products	
Bread, brown, 2 slices	70
white, 2 slices	70
wholemeal, 2 slices	35
1 chapati	20
Milk and dairy products	
½ pint milk, whole, semi-skimmed or skimmed	**350**
½ pint soya milk	50
1 pot yoghurt, plain (150 g)	*300*
fruit (150 g)	*250*
Cheese, Brie (50 g)	*270*
Camembert (50 g)	*175*
Cheddar (50 g)	**360**
Cheddar, reduced fat (50 g)	**420**
Cottage cheese (100 g)	73
Cream cheese (30 g)	35
Edam (50 g)	**350**
Feta (50 g)	*180*
Fromage Frais (100 g)	85
White cheese (50 g)	*280*
1 egg size 2 (60 g)	35
Fish	
Pilchards, canned (105 g)	*105*
Prawns (80 g)	*120*
Salmon, canned (115 g)	100
Sardines, canned (70 g)	**350**
Shrimps (80 g)	100
Whitebait (100 g)	**860**
Vegetables	
Broccoli (100 g)	40
Spinach (100 g)	*150*
Spring greens (100 g)	75
1 small can baked beans (200 g)	106
Dahl, chickpea (150 g)	100
Lentils, kidney beans or chick peas (105 g)	40–70
Soya beans, cooked (100 g)	85
Tofu (60 g)	*300*
Fruit	
1 large orange	70
Nuts and chocolate	
20 almonds	50
1 tablespoon sesame seeds (20 g)	*140*
Tahini paste on 1 slice bread (10 g)	70
Milk chocolate (100 g)	*240*

Excellent source (**bold**). Good source (*italics*).
Information derived from *The Composition of Foods*, 5th Edition (1991) is reproduced with the permission of The Royal Society of Chemistry and the Controller of Her Majesty's Stationery Office.

Metabolism

Absorption
Calcium is absorbed in the duodenum, jejunum and ileum by an active saturable process which involves vitamin D. At high intakes some calcium is absorbed by passive diffusion (independent of vitamin D). It can also be absorbed from the colon.

Distribution
More than 99% of the body's calcium is stored in the bone and teeth. The physiologically active form of calcium is the ionized form (in the blood). Blood calcium levels are controlled homeostatically by parathyroid hormone, calcitonin and vitamin D, and a range of other hormones.

Elimination
Excretion of calcium occurs in the urine, although a large amount is reabsorbed in the kidney tubules, and the amount excreted varies with the quantity of calcium absorbed and the degree of bone loss. Elimination of unabsorbed and endogenously-secreted calcium occurs in the faeces. Calcium is also lost in the sweat and is excreted in breast milk.

Bioavailability
Bioavailability is dependent on vitamin D status. Absorption is reduced by phytates (present in bran and high-fibre cereals), but high-fibre diets at currently recommended levels of intake do not significantly affect calcium absorption in the long term. Absorption is reduced by oxalic acid (present in cauliflower, spinach and rhubarb). High sodium intake may reduce calcium retention.

The efficiency of absorption is increased during periods of high physiological requirement (e.g. in childhood, adolescence, pregnancy and lactation) and impaired in the elderly.

Deficiency
Simple calcium deficiency is not a recognized clinical disorder. Low dietary intake during adolescence and young adulthood may reduce peak bone mass and bone mineral content and increase the risk of osteoporosis in later life.

Uses
Requirements may be increased and/or supplements may be necessary in:

- children, adolescents, pre- and post-menopausal women,
- pregnant and breast-feeding women,
- vegans, and
- lactose intolerance (due to avoidance of milk and milk products).

Osteoporosis
Calcium supplements may have a role in the prevention of osteoporosis. A review (Heaney 1993) identified 43 published studies since 1988 that related calcium intake to bone mass; 26 reported that calcium was positively

correlated with bone mass or inversely related to bone loss or fracture, whereas 16 did not. Inadequate dietary calcium during the critical growth periods may result in failure to reach peak bone mass, leading to increased risk of fracture in later life (Matkovic *et al.* 1990).

Several investigative studies have reported that calcium supplementation attenuates bone loss in peri-menopausal (Elders *et al.* 1991) and menopausal (Dawson-Hughes *et al.* 1990; Reid *et al.* 1993) women. Chapuy *et al.* (1992) showed a reduction in fracture incidence in an elderly population (mean age = 84 years) during a prospective trial of calcium and vitamin D supplementation. These studies show the benefits of calcium supplementation.

Hypertension

Epidemiological studies (Iso *et al.* 1991; McCarron & Morris 1987) support an inverse relationship between the amount of calcium in the diet and blood pressure. However, based on multi-variate analyses, the absolute contribution of calcium is very small. Some clinical intervention studies have reported reduction in blood pressure in normotensive and hypertensive subjects (Grobbee & Hofman 1986; McCarron *et al.* 1990; Singer *et al.* 1985) or no effect (Galloe *et al.* 1993).

In some patients with hypertension and high levels of plasma renin, blood pressure may actually rise in response to calcium supplementation (Resnick *et al.* 1984).

The association between increased calcium intake and lowered blood pressure is suggestive but inconclusive. It is inappropriate to recommend oral calcium supplements for the treatment of hypertension.

Cancer

Calcium may protect against colon cancer. The relationship of calcium intake to colon cancer has been examined in a review of the epidemiological literature (Garland *et al.* 1991), which suggests a protective role of dietary calcium for both colon and rectal cancer. Clinical trials in some high-risk patients (Lipkin *et al.* 1989; Rozen *et al.* 1987) showed a reduction in colonic mucosal proliferation, but another trial (Gregoire *et al.* 1989) did not. Current evidence is inconclusive and further trials are warranted.

Preliminary epidemiological observations (Van 'T Veer *et al.* 1991) suggest an association between calcium intake and protection from breast cancer, but the correlation is weak.

Miscellaneous

There is emerging evidence for a protective role of calcium in hypercholesterolaemia (Sharlin *et al.* 1992) and in diabetes mellitus (Colditz *et al.* 1992). However, calcium supplements should not be recommended for these conditions.

Precautions/contra-indications

Calcium supplements should be avoided in:

- conditions associated with hypercalcaemia and hypercalciuria,

- renal impairment (chronic), and
- renal stones or history of renal stones.

They should be used with caution and with medical supervision in hypertension because blood pressure control may be altered.

Pregnancy and breast-feeding

No problems reported; supplements may be required during pregnancy and lactation.

Adverse effects

Reported adverse effects with supplements include nausea, constipation and flatulence (usually mild). Calcium metabolism is under such tight control that accumulation in blood or tissues from excessive intakes is almost unknown; accumulation is usually due to failure of control mechanisms. Toxic effects and hypercalcaemia are unlikely with oral doses of less than 2000 mg daily. However, in young children, calcium supplements should be used under medical supervision because of a risk of bowel perforation.

Interactions

Drugs

Alcohol: excessive alcohol intake may reduce calcium absorption.
Aluminium-containing antacids: may reduce calcium absorption.
Anticonvulsants: may reduce serum calcium levels.
Bisphosphanates: calcium may reduce absorption of etidronate; give two hours apart.
Cardiac glycosides: concurrent use with parenteral calcium preparations may increase risk of cardiac arrhythmias (ECG monitoring recommended).
Corticosteroids: may reduce serum calcium levels.
Laxatives: prolonged use of laxatives may reduce calcium absorption.
Loop diuretics: increased excretion of calcium.
4-quinolones: may reduce absorption of 4-quinolones and vice-versa; give two hours apart.
Tamoxifen: calcium supplements may increase the risk of hypercalcaemia (a rare side effect of tamoxifen therapy); calcium supplements are best avoided.
Tetracyclines: may reduce absorption of tetracyclines and vice-versa; give two hours apart.
Thiazide diuretics: may reduce calcium excretion.

Nutrients

Fluoride: may reduce absorption of fluoride and vice versa; give two hours apart.
Iron: calcium carbonate or calcium phosphate may reduce absorption of iron; give two hours apart (absorption of iron in multiple formulations containing iron and calcium is not significantly altered).
Vitamin D: increased absorption of calcium and increased risk of hypercalcaemia; may be advantageous in some individuals.
Zinc: may reduce absorption of zinc.

Interference with diagnostic tests
Excessive and prolonged use of calcium may interfere with:

* serum phosphate concentrations (may be decreased).

Dose
Prevention of osteoporosis, post-menopausal women, 1000–1500 mg (as elemental calcium) daily (not a substitute for Hormone Replacement Therapy).

Dietary supplement, up to 1000 mg (as elemental calcium) daily; doses of 2000 mg daily should not be exceeded (when used as a supplement).

Note: doses are given in terms of elemental calcium. Patients should be advised that calcium supplements are not identical; they provide different amounts of elemental calcium. The calcium content of various calcium salts commonly used in supplements is shown in Table 9.1.

Table 9.1 Calcium content of commonly used calcium salts

Calcium Salt	Calcium (mg/g)	Calcium (%)
Calcium amino acid chelate	180	18
Calcium carbonate	400	40
Calcium chloride	272	27.2
Calcium glubionate	65	6.5
Calcium gluconate	90	9
Calcium lactate	130	13
Calcium lactate gluconate	129	13
Calcium orotate	210	21
Calcium phosphate (dibasic)	230	23

Note: Calcium lactate and gluconate are more efficiently absorbed than calcium carbonate (particularly in patients with achlorhydria).

References and further reading
British Nutrition Foundation (1991) *Calcium. BNF Briefing Paper (24).* British Nutrition Foundation, London.

Chapuy M.C., Ariot M.E. & Duboeuf F. (1992) Vitamin D$_3$ and calcium to prevent hip fractures in elderly women. *N Engl J Med* **327**, 1637–42.

Colditz G.A., Manson J.E., Stampfer M.J., Rosner B., Willett W.C. & Speizer F.E. (1992) Diet and risk of clinical diabetes. *Am J Clin Nutr* **55**, 1018–23.

Dawson-Hughes B., Dallal G.E., Krall E.A., Sadowski L., Sahyoun N. & Tannenbaum S. (1990) A controlled trial of the effect of calcium supplementation on bone density in postmenopausal women. *N Engl J Med* **323**, 878–83.

Elders P.J.M., Netelenbos J.C. & Lips P. (1991) Calcium supplementation reduces vertebral bone loss in perimenopausal women; a controlled trial in 248 women between 46 and 55 years of age. *J Clin Endocrinol Metab* **73**, 533–40.

Galloe A.M., Graudal N., Moller J., Bro H., Jorgensen M. & Christensen H.R. (1993) Effect of oral calcium supplementation on blood pressure in patients with previously untreated hypertension: a randomised, double-blind, placebo-controlled, cross-over study. *J Human Hypertension* **7**, 43–5.

Garland C.F., Garland F.C. & Gorham E.D. (1991) Can colon cancer incidence and death rates be reduced with calcium and vitamin D? *Am J Clin Nutr* **54**, 193S–201S.

Gossel T.A. (1991) Calcium Supplements. *US Pharmacist* April, 26–32.

Gregoire R.C., Stern H.S., Yeung K.S., Stadler J., Langley S., Furrer R. & Bruce W.R. (1989) Effect of calcium supplementation on mucosal cell proliferation in high risk patients for colon cancer. *Gut* **30**, 376–82.

Grobbee D.E. & Hofman A. (1986) Effect of calcium supplementation on diastolic blood pressure in young people with mild hypertension. *Lancet* **2**, 703–7.

Heaney R.P. (1993) Nutritional factors in osteoporosis. *Ann Rev Nutr* **13**, 287–316.

Iso H., Terao A. & Kitamura A. (1991) Calcium intake and blood pressure in seven Japanese populations. *Am J Epidemiol* **133**, 776–83.

Li Wan Po A. (1990) Calcium supplements and postmenopausal osteoporosis. *Pharm J* **244**, 117–9.

Lipkin M., Friedman E., Winawer S.J. & Newmark H. (1989) Colonic epithelial cell proliferation in responders and non-responders to supplemental dietary calcium. *Cancer Res* **49**, 248–54.

Matkovic V., Fontana D., Tominac C., Goel P., Chesnut C.H. III. (1990) Factors that influence peak bone mass formation: a study of calcium balance and the inheritance of bone mass in adolescent females. *Am J Clin Nutr* **52**, 878–88.

McCarron D.A. & Morris C.D. (1987) The calcium deficiency hypothesis of hypertension. *Ann Intern Med* **107**, 919–22.

McCarron D.A., Lipkin M., Rivlin R.S. & Heaney R.P. (1990) Dietary calcium and chronic diseases. *Med Hypotheses* **31**, 265–73.

National Dairy Council (1992) *Calcium and Health. Fact File No. 1.* The National Dairy Council, London.

National Osteoporosis Society (1993) *Calcium Guide Book.* National Osteoporosis Society, Bath.

Reid I.R., Ames R.W., Evans M.C., Gamble G.D. & Sharpe S.J. (1993) Effect of calcium supplementation on bone loss in postmenopausal women. *N Engl J Med* **328**, 460–4.

Resnick L.M., Nicholson J.P. & Laragh J.H. (1984) Outpatient therapy of essential hypertension with dietary calcium supplementation. *J Am Coll Cardiol* **3**, 616.

Rozen P., Fireman Z., Wax Y. & Ron E. (1987) Oral calcium suppresses increased colonic mucosal proliferation of persons at risk for colorectal neoplasia. *Gastroenterology* **92**, 1603.

Sharlin J., Posner B.M., Gershoff S.N., Zeitlin M.F. & Berger P.D. (1992) Nutritional and behavioral characteristics and determinants of plasma cholesterol levels in men and women. *J Am Diet Ass* **92**, 434–40.

Singer D.R.J., Markandu N.D., Cappuccio F.P., Beynon G.W., Shore A.C. Smith S.J. & MacGregor G.A. (1985) Does oral calcium lower blood pressure – a double blind study. *J Hypertension* **3**, 661.

Smith R. (ed.) (1990) *Osteoporosis.* Royal College of Physicians, London.

Van 'T Veer P., van Leer E.M. & Rietdijk A. (1991) Combination of dietary factors in relation to breast-cancer occurrence. *Int J Cancer* **47**, 649–53.

Whiting S.J. (1993) Calcium supplements review. *Can Pharm J* **126**, 466–70.

Chapter 10
Carnitine

Description
Carnitine is an amino acid derivative.

Nomenclature
Carnitine is sometimes known as vitamin B_T; it is not an officially recognized vitamin.

Constituents
Carnitine exists as two distinct isomers, L-carnitine (naturally occurring carnitine) and D-carnitine (synthetic carnitine). Dietary supplements contain L-carnitine or a DL-carnitine mixture.

Human requirements
No proof of a dietary need exists. Carnitine is synthesized in sufficient quantities to meet human requirements.

Intakes
The average omnivorous diet is estimated to provide 100–300 mg of carnitine daily.

Dietary sources
Meat and dairy products are the best sources. Fruit, vegetables and cereals are poor sources of carnitine. Carnitine is added to infant milk formulae.

Action
Carnitine has the following physiological functions (Goa & Brogden 1987):

- regulation of long-chain fatty acid transport across cell membranes;
- facilitation of beta-oxidation of long-chain fatty acids and ketoacids; and
- transportation of acyl CoA compounds.

Metabolism
Dietary carnitine is absorbed rapidly from the intestine by both passive and active transport mechanisms. Carnitine is synthesized in the liver, brain and kidney from the essential amino acids, lysine and methionine.

Deficiency
Primary carnitine deficiency is caused by impairment in the membrane transport of carnitine. Symptoms may include:

- chronic muscle weakness (due to muscle carnitine deficiency);

- recurrent episodes of coma and hypoglycaemia (usually in infants and children);
- encephalopathy; and
- cardiomyopathy.

Secondary carnitine deficiency occurs in several inherited disorders of metabolism (especially organic acidurias and disorders of beta-oxidation).

Despite the fact that plant foods are poor sources of carnitine, there is no evidence that vegetarians are deficient in carnitine. Endogenous synthesis prevents deficiencies.

Uses

Ischaemic heart disease
Carnitine may be beneficial in patients with ischaemic heart disease, but only those who have low serum carnitine levels. Orally administered carnitine has been shown to improve symptoms of angina (Cherchi *et al.* 1985) and to reduce anginal attacks and glyceryl trinitrate consumption (Garzya & Amico 1980). Carnitine has also been reported to protect against arrhythmias. While these results are of interest, further evidence is required before the role of carnitine, if any, in the management of heart disease, can be defined.

Hyperlipidaemias
Preliminary studies have demonstrated that L-carnitine may reduce blood cholesterol levels. Oral administration of L-carnitine (3–4 g daily) significantly reduced serum levels of total cholesterol or triglyceride or both, and increased those of HDL cholesterol (Pola *et al.* 1979, 1983; Rossi & Siliprandi 1982).

Athletic performance
There is some evidence that carnitine improves athletic performance (by increasing lipid utilization and conserving glycogen supplies in the muscles). An increase in maximal aerobic power was observed in subjects who received L-carnitine 4 g daily (Angelini *et al.* 1986; Marconi *et al.* 1985). Other studies have yielded conflicting results and further investigation is warranted.

Miscellaneous
Carnitine has been claimed to be of value in myalgic encephalomyelitis and as a slimming aid, but there is no evidence for this.

Precautions/contra-indications
Only L-carnitine should be used. The administration of the D-isomer (including the DL-mixture contained in some supplements) may interfere with the normal function of the L-isomer. Carnitine should not be used in cardiovascular disease without medical supervision.

Pregnancy and breast-feeding
No problems reported but carnitine is probably best avoided during pregnancy.

Adverse effects

Serious toxicity has not been reported. Nausea, vomiting and diarrhoea may occur with high doses. The risk of toxicity is greater with the D-isomer than with L-carnitine (see Precautions); myasthenia has been reported with ingestion of DL-carnitine.

Interactions

Drugs

Anticonvulsants: increased excretion of carnitine.
Pivampicillin: increased excretion of carnitine.
Pivmecillinam: increased excretion of carnitine.

Dose

Not established.

References and further reading

Angelini C., Vergani L., Costa L., Martinuzzi A. & Dunner E. (1986) Clinical study of efficacy of L-carnitine and metabolic observations in exercise physiology. In: *Clinical aspects of human carnitine deficiency* (ed. Borum). Pergamon Press, New York.

Cherchi A., Lai C., Angelino F., Trucco G. & Caponnetto S. (1985) Effects of L-carnitine in exercise tolerance in chronic stable angina: a multicenter, double-blind, randomized placebo controlled crossover study. *Int J Clin Pharmacology, Therapy and Toxicology* **23**, 569–72.

Garyza G. & Amico R.M. (1980) Comparative study on the activity of racemic and laevorotatory carnitine in stable angina pectoris. *Int J Tissue Reactions* **2**, 175–80.

Goa K.L. & Brogden R.N. (1987) *l*-Carnitine. A preliminary review of its pharmacokinetics, and its therapeutic use in ischaemic cardiac disease and primary and secondary carnitine deficiencies in relationship to its role in fatty acid metabolism. *Drugs* **34**, 1–24.

Li Wan Po A. (1990) Carnitine: A Scientifically Exciting Molecule. *Pharm J* **245**, 388–9.

Marconi C., Sassi G., Carpinelli A. & Cerretelli P. (1985) Effects of L-carnitine loading on the aerobic and anaerobic performance of endurance athletes. *European J Appl Physiol* **54**, 131–5.

Pola P., Savi L., Grilli M., Flore R. & Sericchio M. (1979) Carnitine in the therapy of dyslipidemic patients. *Current Therapeutic Research* **27**, 208–16.

Pola P., Tondi P., Dal Lago A., Sericchio M. & Flore R. (1983) Statistical evaluation of long-term *l*-carnitine therapy in hyperlipoproteinaemias. *Drugs under Experimental and Clinical Research* **12**, 925–35.

Rossi C.S. & Silprandi N. (1982) Effect of carnitine on serum HDL-cholesterol: report of two cases. *John Hopkins Medical Journal* **150**, 51–4.

Chapter 11
Carotenoids

Description

Carotenoids are natural pigments found in plants, including fruit and vegetables, giving them their bright colour. About 500 carotenoids have been identified of which 50 have pro-vitamin A activity. All-trans betacarotene is the most active on a weight basis and makes the most important quantitative contribution to human nutrition. Betacarotene is fat soluble.

Nomenclature

The term carotenoids (provitamin A) is a generic term used to describe all carotenoids exhibiting qualitatively the biological activity of betacarotene.

Units

The bioavailability of carotenoids (pro-vitamin A) is not as great as that of retinol (pre-formed vitamin A). Although the absorption and utilization of carotenoids varies, the generally accepted relationship is that 6 µg betacarotene is equivalent to 1 µg retinol.

The amount of betacarotene in dietary supplements may be expressed in terms of micrograms or International Units. One unit of betacarotene is defined as the activity of 0.6 µg betacarotene.

Thus: 1 unit betacarotene = 0.6 µg betacarotene
and: 1 µg betacarotene = 1.67 units betacarotene

Human requirements

There is currently no UK DRV for betacarotene because, until recently, its only role has been considered to be as a precursor of vitamin A. Some authorities are starting to make recommendations for betacarotene, e.g. 6 mg daily (Finland); 4 mg daily (France); 2 mg daily (Germany).

Intakes

In the UK the average adult diet provides 2.28 mg daily.

Action

Betacarotene has the following functions. It:

- acts as a precursor of retinol (pro-vitamin A);
- quenches singlet oxygen and prevents the formation of free radicals;
- reacts with or scavenges free radicals directly and thus acts as an anti-oxidant; and
- enhances some aspects of immune function.

Dietary sources

Food portion	Carotene µg[1]
Bread and cereals	Trace
Milk and dairy products	
Milk	Trace
Cheese – average (50 g)	100
Butter on 1 slice bread (10 g)	40
Margarine on 1 slice bread (10 g)	75
2 tablespoons ghee (30 g)	150
Meat and fish	
Liver, ox, cooked (90 g)	**1400**
Liver, lambs, cooked (90 g)	90
Fish	Trace
Fish oils	Trace
Vegetables	
Peas, boiled, (100 g)	400
Broccoli, boiled (100 g)	470
Brussels sprouts, boiled (100 g)	320
Cabbage, raw, (100 g)	385
Cabbage, boiled (100 g)	210
Carrots, boiled (100 g)	**7560**
Kale, boiled (100 g)	**3375**
Lettuce (30 g)	120
Peppers, green, raw (50 g)	130
Peppers, red, raw, (50 g)	**1920**
Spinach, boiled, (100 g)	**3840**
Sweet potato, boiled, (150 g)	**6000**
2 tomatoes, raw, (150 g)	960
1 large glass tomato juice	400
Watercress (20 g)	500
Mixed vegetable curry (300 g)	**10 200**
Fruit	
1 apple	20
3 apricots	450
1 banana	30
1 mango	**3600**
½ melon, cantaloupe	**2500**
1 slice melon, honeydew	100
1 slice watermelon	750
1 orange	75
4 passion fruits	**1500**
1 slice paw-paw	**1800**
1 peach	90
1 pear	30
3 plums	300

1. To convert carotene (µg) to retinol (µg), divide by 6.
Excellent sources (> 1000 µg/portion) (**bold**).

Metabolism

Absorption

Betacarotene is absorbed into the mucosal cell of the small intestine and converted to retinol. The efficiency of absorption is usually 20–50%, but can be as low as 10% when intake is high. The conversion of betacarotene to retinol is regulated by the vitamin A stores of the individual and by the amount ingested; conversion efficiency varies from 2:1 at low intakes to 12:1 at higher intakes. On average 25% of absorbed betacarotene appears to remain intact and 75% is converted to retinol.

Distribution

Intact betacarotene is transported in very low density lipoprotein (VLDL) or low density lipoprotein (LDL) cholesterol. Blood levels, unlike those of retinol, are not maintained constant; they vary roughly in proportion to the amounts ingested. Increased blood levels (hypercarotenaemia) are sometimes associated (as a secondary condition) with hypothyroidism, diabetes mellitus, and hepatic and renal disease. Hypercarotenaemia can also be caused by a rare genetic inability to convert betacarotene to vitamin A.

Carotenoids are deposited in the liver to a lesser extent than is vitamin A. Most are stored in the adipose tissue, epidermal and dermal layers of the skin and the adrenals; there are high levels in the corpus luteum and in colostrum.

Elimination

Betacarotene is eliminated mainly in the faeces.

Bioavailability

Betacarotene is not very stable. Potency is lost if it is exposed to oxygen. Mild cooking processes can improve bioavailability e.g. absorption from raw carrot can be as low as 1%. This figure increases dramatically when carrots are subject to short periods of boiling. However, overcooking reduces bioavailability. Significant losses can also occur in frying, freezing and canning.

Deficiency

No specific symptoms have been defined.

Uses

Cancer

More than 50 epidemiological studies have demonstrated that a high intake of foods rich in carotenoids (i.e. fruit and vegetables) and high serum levels of betacarotene are associated with reduced risk of certain cancers, especially lung cancer, but also cancers of the cervix, endometrium, breast, oesophagus, mouth and stomach (Gaby & Singh 1991).

Many of these studies report associations with foods rather than betacarotene itself. Fruit and vegetables contain several types of carotenoids in addition to betacarotene. However, serum analysis has shown an association between low serum betacarotene levels and increased cancer risk, possibly indicating a more specific link. Intervention studies published so far (see Section 3) have provided little evidence for a beneficial effect of beta-carotene supplementation on cancer risk. Indeed one study from Finland (The Alpha-Tocopherol, Beta Carotene Cancer Prevention Study Group 1994) showed an increased risk of lung cancer with betacarotene supplementation. Further controlled studies investigating the influence of supplements are needed.

Cardiovascular disease

Diets rich in fruit and vegetables are generally associated with a lower risk of cardiovascular disease but evidence for a direct protective effect of beta-carotene has recently been reported from the Physician's Health Study in America (Gaziano *et al.* 1990). In an analysis of a subgroup of volunteers who had previously had stable angina or coronary revascularization, 50 mg betacarotene on alternate days reduced subsequent coronary events by 50% compared with placebo.

Cataract

Betacarotene may protect against cataract formation. In a retrospective study (Jaques *et al.* 1988), the group with the lowest serum betacarotene levels had over five times the risk of developing cataract as the group with the highest serum levels.

Precautions/contra-indications

Known hypersensitivity to carotenoids.

Pregnancy and breast-feeding

No problems reported.

Adverse effects

Unlike retinol, carotenoids are generally non-toxic. Even when ingested in large amounts, they are not known to cause birth defects or to cause hypervitaminosis A, primarily because efficiency of absorption decreases rapidly as the dose increases and because conversion to vitamin A is not sufficiently rapid to induce toxicity.

Intake of > 30 mg daily (either from commercial supplements or tomato or carrot juice) may lead to hypercarotenaemia which is characterized by a yellowish colouration of the skin (including the palms of the hands and soles of feet), and a very high concentration of carotenoids in the plasma. This is harmless and reversible and gradually disappears when excessive intake of carotenoids is corrected.

Hypercarotenaemia is clearly differentiated from jaundice by the appearance of the whites of the eyes (yellow in hypercarotenaemia but not in jaundice).

Diarrhoea, dizziness and arthralgia may occur occasionally with carotene supplements. Allergic reactions (hay fever and facial swelling), amenorrhoea and leucopenia have been reported rarely.

According to FAO/WHO, intakes up to 5 mg betacarotene/kg body weight are acceptable.

The only serious toxic manifestation of carotenoid intake is canthaxanthin retinopathy which can develop in patients with erythropoietic proto-porphyria and related disorders who are treated with large daily doses (50–100 mg) of canthaxanthin (a derivative of beta-carotene) for long periods.

Interactions
None specifically established (see also Vitamin A, Section 49).

Interference with diagnostic tests
Betacarotene may increase:

• HDL cholesterol levels.

Dose
Dietary supplement, dose not established; dietary supplements provide 6–15 mg (10 000–25 000 units) per dose.

References
The Alpha-Tocopherol, Beta Carotene Cancer Prevention Study Group (1994) The effect of vitamin E and beta carotene on the incidence of lung cancer in male smokers. *New Engl J Med* **330**, 1029–35.

Gaby S.K. & Singh V.N. (1991) Betacarotene. In: *Vitamin intake and health. A scientific review* (eds. S.K. Gaby, A. Bendich, V.N. Singh & L.J. Machlin). Marcel Dekker, New York.

Gaziano J.M., Manson J.E., Ridker P.M., Buring J.E. & Hennekens C.H. (1990) Beta carotene therapy for chronic stable angina. *Circulation* **82**, Suppl III, 201, Abstr. 0796.

Jacques P.F., Hartz S.C., Chylack L.T., Mcgandy R.B. & Sadowski J.A. (1988) Nutritional status in persons with and without senile cataract: blood vitamin and mineral levels. *Am J Clin Nutr* **48**, 152–8.

Chapter 12
Chlorella

Description

Chlorella is a single-celled freshwater alga. It is Japan's most popular health food.

Constituents

Claimed[1] nutrient content of chlorella

Nutrient	per 100 g	per typical dose (3 g)	% RNI[2]
Protein	66 g	2	—
Fat	9 g	0.3 g	—
Carbohydrate	11 g	0.3 g	—
Vitamin A (as betacarotene)	5,500 µg	165 µg	28
Thiamin	2 mg	0.06 mg	8
Riboflavin	7 mg	0.2 mg	24
Niacin	30 mg	0.9 mg	6
Vitamin B_6	1.5 mg	0.05 mg	4
Vitamin B_{12}	134 µg	4 µg	270
Folic acid	25 µg	0.75 µg	0.4
Pantothenic acid	3.0 mg	0.09 mg	—
Biotin	190 µg	6 µg	—
Vitamin C	60 mg	1.8 mg	5
Vitamin E	17 mg	0.5 mg	—
Choline	270 mg	8.1 mg	—
Inositol	190 mg	5.7 mg	—
Calcium	500 mg	15 mg	2
Magnesium	300 mg	9 mg	3
Potassium	700 mg	21 mg	0.6
Phosphorus	1200 mg	36 mg	6.5
Iron	260 mg	8 mg	80
Zinc	70 mg	2 mg	26
Copper	80 µg	2.4 µg	0.2
Iodine	600 µg	18 µg	13

1. Reported on a product label.
2. Reference Nutrient Intake for men aged 19–50 years.

Uses

Claims for chlorella emphasize the importance of its chlorophyll content. However, chlorophyll is a source of energy for plants, but has no known useful function for humans. Chlorella is promoted as a tonic for general health maintenance; it is a useful source of some nutrients (e.g. betacarotene, riboflavin, vitamin B_{12}, iron and zinc – see Constituents). Chlorella is claimed to contain a unique substance called 'Chlorella Growth Factor'.

In addition, chlorella is claimed to be useful in:

- accelerating the healing of wounds and ulcers;
- improving digestion and bowel function;
- stimulating growth and repair to tissues;
- retarding aging;
- strengthening the immune system;
- improving the condition of the hair, skin, teeth and nails;
- treating colds and respiratory infections; and
- removing poisonous substances from the body.

These claims are based largely on anecdote; chlorella has no proven efficacy.

Adverse effects

None reported.

Dose

Not established; dietary supplements recommend 3 g per daily dose.

Chapter 13
Choline

Description

Choline is associated with the B Complex; it is not an officially recognized vitamin. Choline is an active constituent of dietary lecithin.

Human requirements

Choline is an essential nutrient for several mammalian organisms, but its essentiality as a vitamin for humans has not been established. Recent studies, however, suggest that it may be essential (Zeisel et al. 1991).

Intakes

Estimated dietary intake in the UK is 250–500 mg daily. Choline can also be synthesized in the body from phosphatidylethanolamine.

Action

Choline serves as a source of labile methyl groups for transmethylation reactions. It functions as a component of other molecules such as the neurotransmitter acetylcholine, phosphatidylcholine (lecithin) and sphingomyelin, structural constituents of cell membranes and plasma lipoproteins, platelet activating factor and plasmalogen (a phospholipid found in highest concentrations in cardiac muscle membranes).

It is now recognized that lecithin and sphingomyelin participate in signal transduction (Canty & Zeisel 1994), an essential process for cell growth, regulation and function. Animal studies suggest that choline or lecithin deficiency may interfere with this critical process and that alterations in signal transduction may lead to abnormalities such as cancer and Alzheimer's disease.

Dietary sources

Choline is widely distributed in foods (mainly in the form of lecithin). The richest sources of choline are brewer's yeast, egg yolk, liver, wheatgerm, soya beans, kidney and brain. Oats, peanuts, beans and cauliflower contain significant amounts.

Metabolism

Absorption

Some choline is absorbed intact, probably by a carrier-mediated mechanism; some is metabolized by the gastro-intestinal flora to trimethylamine (which produces a fishy odour).

Distribution
Choline is stored in the brain, kidney and liver, primarily as phosphatidyl choline (lecithin) and sphingomyelin.

Elimination
Elimination of choline occurs mainly in the urine.

Deficiency
Dietary choline deficiency occurs in animals, and abnormal liver function, liver cirrhosis and fatty liver may be associated with choline deficiency in humans. Observations in patients on total parenteral nutrition (TPN) have shown a choline-deficient diet to result in fatty infiltration of the liver, hepatocellular damage and liver dysfunction (Sheard 1986; Zeisel 1988).

Uses
Ingestion of choline can affect the concentration of acetylcholine in the brain. Choline has therefore been suggested to be beneficial in patients with diseases related to impaired cholinergic transmission (e.g. tardive dyskinesia, Huntington's chorea, Alzheimer's disease, Gilles de la Tourette, mania, memory impairment and ataxia).

Comparison of studies is often complicated by lack of standardization of doses used. However, clinical trials with tardive dyskinesia patients using choline have met with some success (Davis *et al.* 1975; Gelenberg *et al.* 1979; Growdon *et al.* 1977; Tamminga *et al.* 1977). The efficacy of choline in other disorders has been less convincing.

Claims have been made for the value of choline in the prevention of cardiovacular disease, including angina, atherosclerosis, hypertension, stroke and thrombosis. It has also been claimed to prevent and/or treat Alzheimer's disease, senile dementia and memory loss. Scientific proof for these claims is lacking. More research is needed to clarify the relationship between choline and health and disease states.

Pregnancy and breast-feeding
No problems reported; probably best avoided.

Adverse effects
Fishy odour; more severe symptoms relate to excessive cholinergic transmission (doses of 10 g/d or more) and include:

- diarrhoea,
- nausea,
- dizziness,
- a longer P-R interval in electrocardiograms.

- sweating,
- salivation,
- depression and

Interactions
None established.

Dose
Not established; dietary supplements generally provide 250–500 mg per

dose; (choline chloride provides 80% choline and choline tartrate 50% choline).

References

Canty D.J. & Zeisel S.H. (1994) Lecithin and choline in human health and disease. *Nutr Rev* **52**, 327–39.

Davis K.L., Berger P.A. & Hollister L.E. (1975) Choline for tardive dyskinesia. *New Engl J Med* **293**, 152–3.

Gelenberg A.J., Doller-Wojcik J.C. & Growdon J.H. (1979) Choline and lecithin in the treatment of tardive dyskinesia: preliminary results from a pilot study. *Am J Psychiatr* **136**, 772–6.

Growdon J.H., Hirsch M.J., Wurtman R.J. & Wiener W. (1977) Oral choline administration to patients with tardive dyskinesia. *New Engl J Med* **297**, 524–7.

Sheard N.F., Tayek J.A., Bistrian B.R., Blackburn G.L. & Zeisel S.H. (1986) Plasma choline concentration in humans fed parenterally. *Am J Clin Nutr* **43**, 219–24.

Tamminga C.A., Smith R.C., Erickson S.E., Chang S. & Davis J.M. (1977) Cholinergic influences in tardive dyskinesia. *Am J Psychiatr* **134**, 769–74.

Zeisel S.H. (1988) Vitamin-like molecules. In: *Modern nutrition in health and disease* (eds M.E. Shils & V.R. Young). Lea & Febiger, Philadelphia: pp 440–58.

Zeisel S.H., DaCosta K.A.; Franklin P.D. *et al.* (1991) Choline, an essential nutrient for humans. *FASEB J* **5**, 2093–8.

Chapter 14
Chromium

Description
Chromium is an essential trace mineral.

Human requirements
In the UK no Reference Nutrient Intake or Estimated Average Requirement has been set. A safe and adequate intake is, for adults, 50–400 µg daily; children and adolescents, 0.1–1.0 µg/kg daily.

Intakes
In the UK the average adult diet provides 13.6–47.7 µg daily.

Action
Chromium functions as an organic complex known as glucose tolerance factor (GTF), which is thought to be a complex of chromium, nicotinic acid and amino acids. It potentiates the action of insulin and thus influences carbohydrate, fat and protein metabolism. Chromium also appears to influence nucleic acid synthesis and to play a role in gene expression.

Dietary sources
Wholegrain cereals (including bran cereals), brewer's yeast, processed meats and spices are the best sources. Dairy produce, fruits and vegetables are poor sources.

Metabolism

Absorption
Chromium is poorly absorbed (0.5–2% of intake); absorption occurs in the small intestine by mechanisms which have not been clearly elucidated, but which appear to involve processes other than simple diffusion.

Distribution
Chromium is transported in the serum or plasma bound to transferrin and albumin. It is widely distributed in the tissues.

Elimination
Absorbed chromium is excreted mainly by the kidneys, with small amounts lost in hair, sweat and bile.

Bioavailability
Absorption of chromium is increased by oxalate and by iron deficiency, and reduced by phytate. Diets high in simple sugars (glucose, fructose, sucrose)

increase urinary chromium losses. Absorption is also increased in patients with diabetes mellitus and depressed in the elderly. Stress and increased physical activity appear to increase urinary losses.

Deficiency

Gross chromium deficiency is rarely seen in humans, but signs and symptoms of marginal deficiency include:

- impaired glucose intolerance,
- fasting hyperglycaemia,
- raised circulating insulin levels,
- glycosuria,
- decreased insulin binding,
- reduced number of insulin receptors,
- elevated serum cholesterol,
- elevated serum triglycerides, and
- central and peripheral neuropathy.

Uses

Chromium is claimed to be a useful supplement for diabetic patients and to reduce blood cholesterol levels.

Glucose metabolism

It decreases blood sugar in individuals with elevated blood glucose and may also lead to increases in blood glucose in individuals with low blood sugar (Anderson *et al.* 1983). Both of these effects relate to normalization of insulin and possibly to an increase in the number of insulin receptors.

Supplemental chromium was shown to improve hypoglycaemic symptoms, blood glucose values and insulin receptor number in a study of eight hypoglycaemic female patients (Anderson *et al.* 1987) and to improve blood glucose values and hypoglycaemic symptoms in a study of 20 patients (Clausen 1988), but not all studies have shown beneficial effects.

The possibility that chromium deficiency is responsible for some cases of impaired glucose and insulin metabolism cannot be ignored, but there is insufficient evidence to make claims for the need for dietary supplements.

Cardiovascular disease

Chromium deficiency has been suggested as a risk factor for cardiovascular disease (Simonoff 1984). Supplemental chromium has been shown to increase HDL cholesterol and decrease total cholesterol in some studies (Wallach 1985), but not in others (Anderson *et al.* 1983; Rabinowitz *et al.* 1983).

Miscellaneous

Physical trauma (Borel *et al.* 1984) and strenuous exercise (Anderson *et al.* 1984) lead to increased urinary chromium losses, but the significance of these findings on chromium status is not clear. Chromium has also been promoted as a slimming aid on the basis that it increases the metabolic rate but these claims have not been substantiated.

Precautions/contra-indications

Chromium supplements containing yeast should be avoided by patients taking monoamine oxidase inhibitors (MAOIs). Patients with diabetes mellitus should not take chromium supplements unless medically supervised.

Pregnancy and breast-feeding

No problems reported at normal intakes.

Adverse effects

Oral chromium, particularly trivalent chromium (the usual form in supplements), is relatively non-toxic and unlikely to induce adverse effects. Industrial exposure to high amounts of chromate dust is associated with an increased incidence of lung cancer and may cause allergic dermatitis and skin ulcers. The hexavalent form (not found in food or supplements) can cause renal and hepatic necrosis.

Interactions

Drugs

Insulin: may reduce insulin requirements in diabetes mellitus (monitor blood glucose).
Oral hypoglycaemics: may potentiate effects of oral hypoglycaemics.

Interference with diagnostic tests

Chromium may interfere with:

- blood glucose concentrations (decrease), and
- glucose tolerance tests.

Dose

Not established; dietary supplements provide, on average, 200 µg daily.

References

Anderson R.A., Polansky M.M., Bryden N.A., Roginski E.E., Mertz W. & Glinsmann W. (1983) Chromium supplementation of human subjects: effects on glucose, insulin and lipid variables. *Metabolism* **32**, 894–9.

Anderson R.A., Polansky M.M. & Bryden N.A. (1984) Strenuous running. Acute effects of chromium, copper, zinc and selected clinical variables in urine and serum of male runners. *Biol Trace Elem Res* **6**, 327–36.

Anderson R.A., Polansky M.M., Bryden N.A., Bhathena S.J. & Canary J (1987) Effects of supplemental chromium on patients with symptoms of reactive hypoglycaemia. *Metabolism* **36**, 351–5.

Borel J.S., Majerus T.C., Polansky M.M., Moser P.B. & Anderson R.A. (1984) Chromium intake and urinary chromium excretion of trauma patients. *Biol Trace Elem Res* **6**, 317–26.

Clausen J. (1988) Chromium induced clinical improvement in symptomatic hypoglycaemia. *Biol Trace Elem Res* **17**, 229–36.

Rabinowitz M.B., Gonick H.C., Levin S.R. & Davidson M.B. (1983) Clinical trial of chromium and yeast supplements on carbohydrate and lipid metabolism in diabetic men. *Biol Trace Elem Res* **5**, 449–66.

Simonoff M. (1984) Chromium deficiency and cardiovascular disease. *Cardiovasc Res* **18**, 591–6.
Wallach S. (1985) Clinical and biochemical aspects of chromium deficiency. *J Am Coll Nutr* **4**, 107–20.

Chapter 15
Coenzyme Q

Description
Coenzyme Q is a naturally occurring enzyme (found in the mitochondria of body cells).

Nomenclature
Alternative names include coenzyme Q10 and ubiquinone.

Action
Coenzyme Q is involved in electron transport in the mitochondrial membrane. It is important for energy production in cells, is thought to be a free radical scavenger, an antioxidant and to have membrane stabilizing properties.

Dietary sources
The coenzyme Q content of different types of food has been evaluated by Kamei *et al*. (1986). Coenzyme Q is found in fatty fish (such as sardines and mackerel), wholegrain cereals, soya beans, nuts, meat and poultry, and vegetables (especially spinach and broccoli). Milk and cheese have a lower content of coenzyme Q.

Endogenous synthesis is also important and the relative importance of biosynthesis and dietary intake to coenzyme Q status has not been clarified.

Metabolism
Coenzyme Q is synthesized endogenously using tyrosine, methionine and acetyl CoA as starting materials. The acetyl CoA pathway proceeds to both cholesterol and coenzyme Q synthesis, so coenzyme Q10 and cholesterol share, to some extent, the same biosynthetic pathway.

The ability to synthesize coenzyme Q may decrease with age. Evidence for a reduction in coenzyme Q10 concentrations with age in various human tissues has been demonstrated (Kalen *et al*. 1989; Soderberg *et al*. 1990).

Uses

Cardiovascular disease
Coenzyme Q has been suggested to have a role in the management of cardiovascular disease. A study in Italy investigated the effects of coenzyme Q used as an adjunct to conventional treatment in 2500 patients. Improvement in major clinical symptoms such as cyanosis, oedema and arrhythmias emerged from preliminary results in 1113 patients (Baggio *et al*. 1993). In a long-term placebo controlled study by Morisco *et al*. (1993), in which coenzyme Q 2 mg/kg was given to 319 heart failure patients,

hospital admission rates and symptom severity were significantly reduced.

Langsjoen *et al.* (1990) concluded from a six-year study that coenzyme Q was a safe and effective long-term treatment for chronic cardiomyopathy. Use of coenzyme Q in patients undergoing cardiac surgery has demonstrated a therapeutic benefit in preserving myocardial integrity (Judy *et al.* 1993).

Cancer

Coenzyme Q is claimed to have a protective effect against cancer. Folkers *et al.* (1993) reported that coenzyme Q has shown macrophage potentiating activity in cancer patients with some evidence of increased survival. In a Danish trial (Lockwood *et al.* 1994) 32 women were given routine chemotherapy, radiotherapy, surgery, vitamins, minerals and coenzyme Q. Six of the women showed partial or complete cancer regression. The authors concluded that, statistically, six women would normally have died, but during the two years of the trial there were no deaths. However, the multiplicity of nutritional supplements used in the study prevents identification of coenzyme Q as the dominant factor.

Miscellaneous

Trials have shown beneficial effects of coenzyme Q in gingivitis. Hanioka *et al.* (1993) reported that coenzyme Q could stop gum bleeding and anchor loose teeth.

Several other claims have been made for coenzyme Q including improved energy levels, reduced menopausal symptoms, improved immunity, reduced blood pressure and as an aid to slimming, but there is limited evidence for these claims.

Results from preliminary studies with coenzyme Q justify more rigorous trials to investigate potential benefits, but there is insufficient evidence to make definite recommendations for coenzyme Q as a dietary supplement.

Precautions/contra-indications

Coenzyme Q should not be used to treat cardiovascular disorders without medical supervision.

Pregnancy and breast-feeding

No problems reported; probably best avoided.

Adverse effects

No adverse effects have been reported except for occasional, mild nausea. Withdrawal of coenzyme Q could cause relapse in patients with cardiovascular disorders.

Interactions

Warfarin: may reduce the effect of warfarin; decreases in international normalized ratio (INR) have been reported (Spigset 1994).

Dose

Not established; as an adjunct to conventional treatment in cardiovascular disorders (with medical supervision only), doses of 150–300 mg daily have been used; dietary supplements generally provide 15–60 mg per dose.

References and further reading

Baggio E., Gandini R., Plancher C., Passeri N. & Carmosino G. (1993) Italian multi-centre study of the efficacy and safety of Q10 as adjuvant therapy in heart failure (interim analysis). *Clin Invest* **71**, S145–9.

Folkers K., Brown R., Judy W.V. & Morita M. (1993) Survival of cancer patients on therapy with coenzyme Q10. *Biochem Biophys Res Commun* **192**, 241–5.

Greenberg S. & Frishman W.H. (1990). Coenzyme Q_{10}: a new drug for cardiovascular disease. *J Clin Pharmacol* **30**, 596–608.

Hanioka T., McRee J., Xia L. & Folkers K. (1993) Biochemical evidence supporting effective therapy with CoQ10 for subgingival micro-organisms in periodontal disease. *Proc 8th Int Symp on Q10, Stockholm.*

Judy W.V., Stogsdill W.W. & Folkers K. (1993) Myocardial preservation by therapy with coenzyme Q10 during heart surgery. *Clin Invest* **71**, S155–61.

Kalen A., Appelkvist E.L. & Dallner G. (1989) Age related changes in the lipid composition of rat and human tissue. *Lipids* **24**, 579–84.

Kamei M., Fujita T., Ranke T., Sasaki K., Ohiba K., Otani S., Matsui-Yuasa T. & Morisawa S. (1986) The distribution and content of ubiquinone in foods. *International J Vit Nutr Res* **56**, 57–64.

Langsjoen P.H., Folkers K., Lyson K., Muratusu K., Lyson T. & Langsjoen P. (1990) Pronounced increase of survival of patients with cardiomyopathy when treated with coenzyme Q10 and conventional therapy. *Int J Tissue React* **12**, 163–8.

Lockwood K., Moesgaard S., Hanioka T. & Folkers K. (1994) Apparent partial remission of breast cancer in 'high risk' patients supplemented with nutritional antioxidants, essential fatty acids and coenzyme Q10. *Biochem Biophys Res Commun* **199**, 1504–8.

Morisco C., Trimarco B. & Condorelli M. (1993) Effect of coenzyme Q10. Therapy in patients with congestive heart failure: a long term multicenter randomized study. *Clin Invest* **71**, S134–6.

Soderberg M., Edlund C., Kristensson K. & Dallner G. (1990) Lipid composition of different regions of the brain during aging. *J Neurochem* **54**, 415–23.

Spigset O. (1994) Reduced effect of warfarin caused by ubidecarone. *Lancet* **344**, 1372–1373.

Chapter 16
Copper

Description
Copper is an essential trace mineral.

Human requirements
Dietary Reference Values (mg/d)

Age	RNI
0–12 months	0.3
1–3 years	0.4
4–6 years	0.6
7–10 years	0.7
11–14 years	0.8
15–16 years	1.0
18–50+ years	1.2
Pregnancy	1.2
Lactation	1.5

Note: No EAR or LRNI have been derived for copper.
Reproduced and adapted with the permission of the Controller of Her Majesty's Stationery Office.

Intakes
In the UK the average adult diet provides: for men, 1.82 mg daily; for women, 1.31 mg.

Action
Copper functions as an essential component of many enzymes and other proteins. It plays a role in bone formation and mineralization, and in the integrity of the connective tissue of the cardiovascular system. Copper is involved in iron metabolism, melanin pigment formation, cholesterol metabolism and glucose metabolism. In the central nervous system, it is required for the formation of myelin and is important for normal neurotransmission. Copper has pro-oxidant effects *in vitro* but antioxidant effects *in vivo* and there is accumulating evidence that adequate copper is required to maintain antioxidant effects within the body (Strain 1994).

Dietary sources

Food portion	Copper content (mg)
Breakfast cereals	
1 bowl All-Bran (45 g)	*0.2*
1 bowl Bran Flakes (45 g)	0.1
1 bowl Muesli (95 g)	*0.3*
2 pieces Shredded Wheat	*0.2*
2 Weetabix	*0.2*
Cereal products	
Bread, brown, 2 slices	0.1
white, 2 slices	0.1
wholemeal 2 slices	*0.2*
1 chapati	0.1
Pasta, brown, boiled (150 g)	*0.3*
white, boiled (150 g)	0.1
Rice, brown, boiled (165 g)	*0.5*
white, boiled (165 g)	*0.2*
Meat	
Meat, average, cooked (100 g)	*0.2*
Liver, lambs, cooked (90 g)	**9.0**
calf, cooked (90 g)	**11.0**
Kidney, lambs, cooked (75 g)	*0.4*
Vegetables	
Chick peas, lentils, or red kidney beans, cooked (105 g)	*0.2*
Potatoes, boiled (150 g)	0.1
Mushrooms, cooked (100 g)	*0.4*
Green vegetables (100 g)	0.02
Fruit	
1 banana	*0.3*
1 orange	0.1
2 handfuls raisins	0.1
8 dried apricots	*0.2*
Nuts and chocolate	
20 almonds	*0.2*
10 Brazil nuts	*0.4*
30 Hazel nuts	*0.4*
30 peanuts	*0.3*
Milk chocolate (100 g)	*0.3*
Plain chocolate (100 g)	**0.7**

Excellent sources (**bold**); good sources (*italic*).
Information derived from *The Composition of Foods*, 5th Edition (1991) is reproduced with the permission of The Royal Society of Chemistry and the Controller of Her Majesty's Stationery Office.

Metabolism

Absorption
Copper is absorbed mainly in the small intestine, with a small amount absorbed in the stomach; absorption is probably by a saturable carrier-mediated mechanism at low levels of intake and by passive diffusion at high levels of intake.

Distribution
Copper is rapidly taken up by the liver and incorporated into caeruloplasmin. It is stored primarily in the liver. Copper is transported bound to caeruloplasmin.

Elimination
Elimination is mainly via bile into the faeces; small amounts are excreted in the urine, sweat and via epidermal shedding.

Bioavailability
Absorption may be reduced by phytate (present in bran and high-fibre foods) and non-starch polysaccharides (dietary fibre), but recommended intakes of fibre-containing foods are unlikely to compromise copper status.

Deficiency
Deficiency of copper may lead to:

- hypochromic and microcytic anaemias,
- leucopenia,
- neutropenia,
- impaired immunity, and
- bone demineralization.

Deficiency may also be caused by Menke's syndrome (an X-linked genetic disorder in which copper absorption is defective); this disease is characterized by

- a reduced level of copper in the blood, liver and hair,
- progressive mental deterioration,
- defective keratinization of the hair, and hypothermia.

Marginal deficiency may result in:

- elevated cholesterol levels,
- impaired glucose tolerance,
- defects in pigmentation and structure of the hair, and
- demyelination and degeneration of the nervous system.

In infants and children, copper deficiency can lead to skeletal fragility and increased susceptibility to infections, especially those of the respiratory tract.

Copper deficiency has been linked to many of the processes, including atherosclerosis and thrombosis, associated with ischaemic heart disease (for review, see Strain 1994). Whether this relationship is important in humans remains unanswered. More information is required concerning possible mild copper deficiency in human populations.

Uses

Copper has been claimed to be protective against hypercholesterolaemia. In various animal species it has been demonstrated that feeding a copper deficient diet results in increased serum cholesterol levels (Klevay *et al.* 1984), but studies in humans have shown inconsistent results (Klevay *et al.* 1984; Medeiros *et al.* 1983; Shapcott *et al.* 1985).

Claims for the value of copper supplements in rheumatoid arthritis and psoriasis have not been proved.

Precautions/contra-indications

Wilson's disease (disorder may be exacerbated); hepatic and biliary disease.

Pregnancy and breast-feeding

No problems reported with normal intakes.

Adverse effects

With excessive doses (unlikely from supplements):

- epigastric pain, anorexia, nausea, vomiting and diarrhoea;
- hepatic toxicity and jaundice;
- hypotension;
- haematuria (blood in urine, pain on urination, lower back pain);
- metallic taste; and
- convulsions and coma.

Copper toxicity may also occur in patients with Wilson's disease (an inherited disorder in which patients exhibit a deficiency of plasma caeruloplasmin and an excess of copper in the liver and bloodstream). There is a theoretical possibility of copper toxicity in women who use copper-containing intra-uterine contraceptive devices (further studies required).

Interactions

Drugs

Penicillamine: reduces absorption of copper and vice versa; give two hours apart.
Trientine: reduces absorption of copper and vice versa; give two hours apart.

Nutrients

Iron: large doses of iron may reduce copper status and vice versa; give two hours apart.
Vitamin C: large doses of vitamin C (> 1 g daily) may reduce copper status.
Zinc: large doses of zinc may reduce absorption of copper and vice versa; give two hours apart.

Dose

Dietary supplement, up to 3 mg (elemental copper) daily. Copper content of various commonly used salts is:

- copper amino acid chelate (20 mg/g);

- copper gluconate (140 mg/g); and
- copper sulphate (254 mg/g).

References
Klevay L.M., Inman L., Johnson L.K., Lawler M., Mahalco J.R., Milne D.B., Lukaski H.C., Bolonchuk W. & Sandstead H.H. (1984) Increased cholesterol in plasma in a young man during experimental copper depletion. *Metabolism* **33**, 1112–8.

Medeiros D., Pellum L. & Brown B. (1983) Serum lipids and glucose as associated with haemoglobin levels and copper and zinc intake in young adults. *Life Sci* **32**, 1897–1904.

Shapcott D., Vobecky J.S., Vobecky J. & Demers P.P. (1985) Plasma cholesterol and the plasma copper/zinc ratio in young children. *Sci Total Environ* **42**, 197–200.

Strain J.J. (1994) Newer aspects of micronutrients in chronic disease: copper. *Proc Nutr Soc* **53**, 583–98.

Chapter 17
Dolomite

Description

Dolomite is normally obtained from limestone

Constituents

The main constituents are calcium and magnesium carbonates.

Uses

As a source of calcium and magnesium.

Precautions/contra-indications

Dolomite may be contaminated with toxic trace elements such as antimony, arsenic, cadmium, lead and mercury (Robert 1983). Supplements are best avoided.

Pregnancy and breast-feeding

Avoid (contaminants – see Precautions).

Adverse effects

None (except contaminants – see Precautions).

Interactions

See calcium (Chapter 9) and magnesium (Chapter 34).

Dose

Dietary supplements provide 250–500 mg calcium and 150–300 mg magnesium per dose.

References

Robert S.H.J. (1983) Potential toxicity due to dolomite and bonemeal. *South Med J* **76**, 556–9.

Chapter 18
Evening Primrose Oil

Description
Evening primrose oil is derived from the seeds of *Oenothera biennis* and other species.

Constituents
Evening primrose oil contains gamma-linolenic acid (GLA) and linoleic acid. Starflower oil (borage oil) and oil of javanicus are also used as sources of GLA in dietary supplements. Evening primrose oil contains 8–11% GLA. Starflower oil contains 20–25% GLA, but the biological activity of starflower oil may be no greater than that of evening primrose oil, i.e. on a weight for weight basis starflower oil has not been proved to be twice as active as evening primrose oil.

Action
GLA is not an essential dietary component. It is normally synthesized in the body by the action of delta-6-desaturase on linoleic acid (obtained in the diet from vegetable and seed oils e.g. sunflower oil).

GLA is a precursor of dihomogamma-linolenic acid (DGLA) and the series 1 prostaglandins, and also of arachidonic acid (see Figure 18.1). Most of the DGLA formed from GLA is metabolised to PG1s; conversion of DGLA to arachidonic acid is very slow. Arachidonic acid is normally obtained from meat in the diet.

Supplementation with GLA increases the ratio of DGLA to arachidonic acid. DGLA levels are elevated to a greater extent by the administration of GLA than by the administration of linoleic acid (although the reasons for this are not entirely clear).

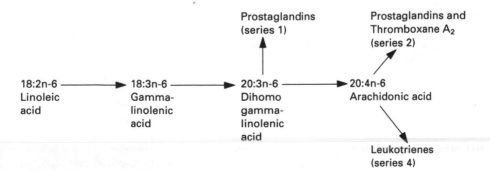

Figure 18.1 Metabolism of gamma-linolenic acid and arachidonic acid

Prostaglandin PGE_1 (produced from DGLA) inhibits platelet aggregation and is also a vasodilator; it has less potent inflammatory effects than prostaglandins of the PG2 series, Thromboxane A_2 and series 4 leukotrienes (produced from arachidonic acid).

The efficacy of GLA is thus thought to be due, in part, to the increased production of PG1 series prostaglandins at the expense of PG2 series prostaglandins, Thromboxane A_2 and series 4 leukotrienes.

Deficiency

Patients with diabetes mellitus or eczema may be at risk of GLA deficiency. Despite some claims, however, there is little evidence that foods rich in saturated fat and sugar, alcohol, stress, pollution, high blood cholesterol, ageing, viral infections and hormone imbalances lead to deficiency of GLA.

Uses

Evening primrose oil is used widely as a dietary supplement for various disorders, including the pre-menstrual syndrome, hypertension, asthma and angina. It is claimed to reduce blood cholesterol levels and to act as a slimming aid.

Disorders for which evening primrose oil has been tested in controlled clinical trials include:

- atopic dermatitis,
- diabetic neuropathy,
- mastalgia and breast cysts,
- menopausal flushing,
- Raynaud's phenomenon,
- rheumatoid arthritis,
- schizophrenia,
- Sjogren's syndrome,
- ulcerative colitis, and
- various cancers.

Evening primrose oil is being investigated in a range of other disorders including multiple sclerosis and hyperactivity in children.

Dermatitis

For atopic dermatitis, Wright & Burton (1982) reported positive effects from a double-blind crossover trial of evening primrose oil in 99 patients, but two other studies (Bamford *et al.* 1985; Berth-Jones & Graham-Brown 1993) reported negative effects. One GLA product is available on the NHS for alleviation of symptoms of eczema; any effect is thought to be modest.

Pre-menstrual syndrome and the menopause

Evening primrose oil appears to help some women with pre-menstrual syndrome. Four clinical trials have shown positive results but Khoo *et al.* (1993) found no differences between placebo and evening primrose oil in a trial of 38 women. In mastalgia and breast tenderness, trials with evening primrose oil have shown positive results (Mansel *et al.* 1990). In a study of 56 post-menopausal women suffering hot flushes (Chenoy *et al.* 1994) gamma-linolenic acid offered no benefit over the placebo.

Rheumatoid arthritis

Results from trials in rheumatoid arthritis have been mixed. In one study of 20 patients, treatment with non-steroidal anti-inflammatory drugs was stopped and administration of evening primrose oil resulted in no significant changes in symptoms of arthritis (Hansen *et al*. 1983). In another study (Belch *et al*. 1988) treatment with evening primrose oil allowed 12 out of 16 patients to stop taking non-steroidal anti-inflammatory drugs. However, other studies have demonstrated no beneficial effects.

Miscellaneous

Encouraging findings have been reported with trials of evening primrose oil in diabetic neuropathy (Jamal & Carmichael 1990; the Gamma Linolenic Acid Multicenter Trial Group 1993).

There is currently no justification for the use of evening primrose oil in asthma, hypertension, coronary heart disease or as a slimming aid.

Precautions/contra-indications

Avoid in patients with epilepsy (small risk) and in those taking epileptogenic drugs, e.g. phenothiazines.

Pregnancy and breast-feeding

Caution in pregnancy (possible hormonal effects). Safe during breast-feeding.

Adverse effects

Toxicity appears to be low. The only adverse effects reported are nausea, diarrhoea and headache. However, one report (Phinney 1994) has warned of a potential risk of inflammation, thrombosis and immunosuppression due to slow accumulation of tissue arachidonic acid after prolonged use of gamma linolenic acid for more than one year.

Interactions

Phenothiazines: increased risk (small) of epileptic fits.

Dose

Symptomatic relief of eczema, 320–480 mg (as GLA) daily; child 1–12 years, 160–320 mg daily.

Symptomatic relief of cyclical and non-cyclical mastalgia, 240–320 mg (as GLA) daily for 12 weeks (then stopped if no improvement).

Dietary supplements provide 40–300 mg (as GLA) per daily dose.

Note: evening primrose oil supplements are not identical; they provide different amounts of GLA.

References

Bamford J.T., Gibson R.W. & Renier C.M. (1985) Atopic eczema unresponsive to evening primrose oil. *J Am Acad Dermatol* **13**, 959–65.

Belch J.J., Ansell D., Madhock R., O'Dowd A. & Sturrock R.D. (1988) The effects of altering dietary essential fatty acids on requirements for non-steroidal anti-inflammatory drugs in patients with rheumatoid arthritis. *Ann Rheum Dis* **47**, 96–104.

Berth-Jones J. & Graham-Brown R.A.C. (1993) Placebo-controlled trial of essential fatty acid supplementation in atopic dermatitis. *Lancet* **341**, 1557–60.

Chenoy S., Hussain S., Tayob Y., O'Brien P.M.S, Moss M.Y., Morse P.F. (1994) Effect of oral gamolenic acid from evening primrose oil on menopausal flushing. *Br Med J* **308**, 501–3.

Gamma-Linolenic Acid Multicenter Trial Group (1993) Treatment of diabetic neuropathy with gamma-linolenic acid. *Diabetes Care* **16**, 8–15.

Hansen T.M., Lerche A., Kassis V., Lorenzen I. & Sondergaard J. (1983) Treatment of rheumatoid arthritis with prostaglandin E1 precursors cis-linoleic acid and gamma-linolenic acid. *Scan J Rheumatol* **12**, 85–8.

Jamal G.A. & Carmichael H. (1990) The effect of gamma-linolenic acid on human diabetic peripheral neuropathy: a double-blind placebo-controlled trial. *Diabetic Medicine* **7**, 319–23.

Khoo S.K., Munro C. & Battistutta D. (1990) Evening primrose oil and treatment of pre-menstrual syndrome. *Med J Austr* **153**, 189–92.

Mansel R.E., Pye J.K. & Hughes L.E. (1990) Effects of essential fatty acids on cyclical mastalgia and non-cyclical breast disorders. In: *Omega-6 essential fatty acids. Pathophysiology and roles in clinical medicine* (ed. D.F. Horrobin), pp 557–66. Wiley-Liss, New York.

Phinney S. (1994) Potential risk of prolonged gamma-linolenic acid use. *Ann Intern Med* **120**, 692.

Wright S. & Burton J.L. (1982) Oral evening primrose seed oil improves atopic eczema. *Lancet* **2**, 120–2.

Chapter 19
Fish Oils

Description
There are two types of fish oil supplements:

1. Fish liver oil; this is generally obtained from the liver of the cod, halibut or shark.
2. Fish body oil; this is normally derived from the flesh of the herring, sardine or anchovy.

Constituents
Fish liver oil is a rich source of vitamins A and D; concentrations in cod liver oil liquids normally range between 750 and 1200 µg (2500–4000 units) vitamin A per 10 ml and 2.5–10 µg (100–400 units) vitamin D per 10 ml; halibut and shark liver oils are more concentrated sources of these vitamins. Fish body oil is low in vitamins A and D. Vitamin E is also present in both types of fish oil and extra vitamin E is normally added to supplements.

Both fish liver oil and fish body are sources of polyunsaturated fatty acids of the omega 3 series (eicosapentaenoic acid (EPA) and docosahexaenoic acid (DHA)).

Human requirements
EPA and DHA can be synthesized in the body (in small amounts) from alpha-linolenic acid (contained in vegetable oils e.g. soyabean, linseed and rape-seed oils). However, there may, in addition, be a small dietary requirement (more evidence is required).

Dietary sources
Fatty fish is the best source, but fried or processed fatty fish (e.g. smoked or pickled) is best avoided.

Approximate EPA/DHA content of fish

Fish	Total EPA/DHA (mg/serving)
Cod	600
Haddock	550
Herring	1500
Mackerel	2500
Plaice	500
Salmon	1600
Sardines	1000
Tuna	500

Action

Fish oils produce several effects (see review – Sanders 1993). These include the following.

1. *Alteration of lipoprotein metabolism.* In both normolipidaemic and hyperlipidaemic subjects fish oils reduce plasma triglycerides and very low density lipoproteins (VLDL) (Harris 1989; Sanders *et al.* 1989; Schmidt *et al.* 1993). With moderate intakes of fish oils both high density lipoproteins (HDL) and low density lipoproteins (LDL) tend to increase. High intakes reduce HDL cholesterol and may increase LDL in some patients.

2. *Inhibition of atherosclerosis.* Atherosclerosis is reported to be rare in Eskimos on their traditional diets of fish and seal, and fish oils inhibit the development of atherosclerosis in animals (Parks *et al.* 1990). Fish oils reduce the plasma concentrations of several atherogenic lipoproteins (see above), but other mechanisms may be important. Omega-3 fatty acids have been shown to reduce vasoconstriction in humans (Chin *et al.* 1993; Kenny *et al.* 1992). This may in part be due to the production of endothelial derived releasing factors (EDRF) (Vanhoutte *et al.* 1991).

3. *Alteration of thrombolysis.* Fish oils have been reported to increase, reduce or have no effect on the dissolution of fibrin in a blood clot.

4. *Prolongation of bleeding time.* Studies have shown consistently that fish oils prolong bleeding time. Several factors control bleeding time and some of these are influenced by fish oils while others are not. Fish oils may reduce platelet adhesiveness to the vascular endothelium. They appear to reduce the tendency of platelets to aggregate (Fumeron *et al.* 1991), but the effect is mild compared with aspirin.

5. *Inhibition of inflammation.* Diets rich in omega-3 fatty acids appear to reduce the inflammatory response (Terano *et al.* 1986).

6. *Inhibition of the immune response.* Immune reactivity is generally reduced by omega-3 fatty acids (Endres *et al.* 1991; Meydani *et al.* 1993).

7. *Inhibition of tumour growth.* Many studies have shown a significant reduction in the growth of transplantable mammary tumours (both in humans and rats) when the animals were fed diets rich in omega-3 fatty acids (Cave 1991). In a double blind, placebo-controlled study of 20 patients with adenomatous colo-rectal polyps, Anti *et al.* (1992) showed that fish oil reduced rectal mucosal proliferation after two weeks of treatment. In a study of 12 patients with breast cancer who received fish oil (Holroyde *et al.* 1988), a measurable clinical response was observed in two patients.

8. *DHA appears to have an important physiological function in the retina* (and hence the visual process). Abnormal retinograms have been found in animals deprived of omega-3 fatty acids (Neuringer *et al.* 1988).

9. *Duration of pregnancy may be prolonged.* Fish oil supplements have been found to prolong gestation in women (Olsen *et al.* 1992) without any obvious adverse effects on the outcome of pregnancy.

Omega-3 fatty acids appear to act by:

- modulation of pro-inflammatory and pro-thrombotic eicosanoid (prostaglandin, thromboxane and leukotriene) production, and
- reduction in interleukin-1 and other cytokines.

Eicosanoid production

The effects of omega-3 fatty acids are thought to be due to the partial replacement of arachidonic acid with EPA in cell membrane lipids. This leads to increased production of PG3 series prostaglandins, thromboxane A_3 and series 5 leukotrienes at the expense of PG2 series prostaglandins, thromboxane A_2 and series 4 leukotrienes (see Figure 19.1).

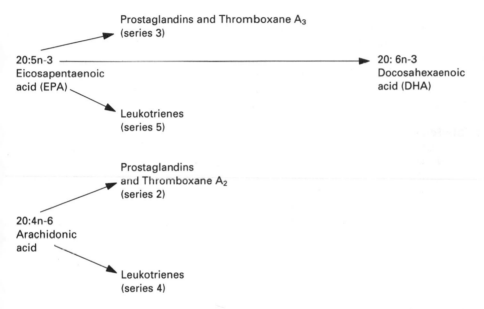

Figure 19.1 Metabolism of eicosapentaenoic acid and arachidonic acid

Thromboxane A_3 (produced from EPA) is weaker at stimulating platelet aggregation than thromboxane A_2 (produced from arachidonic acid). Prostaglandins of the PG3 series have less potent inflammatory effects than prostaglandins of the PG2 series. In addition, DHA inhibits the formation of the more inflammatory prostaglandins of the PG2 series, while EPA acts as a substrate for the synthesis of the less inflammatory prostaglandins of the PG3 series.

Series 5 leukotrienes (produced by EPA) have weaker inflammatory effects than series 4 leukotrienes (produced by arachidonic acid).

Uses

Fish liver oils are used as a source of vitamins A and D. Both fish liver oils and fish body oils are used as a source of EPA and DHA.

Cardiovascular disease

Clinical studies investigating the effects of fish oils in the prevention and treatment of cardiovascular disease are beginning to emerge. A study investigating omega-3 fatty acids in the secondary prevention of myocardial infarction (Burr *et al.* 1989) showed a reduction in total deaths, but total coronary events were not reduced, owing to an increase in non-fatal acute myocardial infarction. These findings offer some promise, but need confirmation.

The use of glyceryl trinitrate in angina was reduced in 12 patients with angina after nine months supplementation with fish oils (Saynor *et al.* 1984), but later studies have been unable to confirm any effects of fish oils on the symptoms of angina (Kristensen *et al.* 1987; Mehta *et al.* 1988).

Some evidence for an anti-arrhythmic effect of fish oils has come from animal studies, but in humans little or no anti-arrhythmic effect has been demonstrated (Christensen *et al.* 1993; Hardarson *et al.* 1989).

Supplements of EPA and DHA have led to modest reductions in blood pressure (3–5 mm Hg in systolic and diastolic pressure) in both normotensive and mildly hypertensive individuals (Bonna *et al.* 1990; Kestin *et al.* 1990), while no effect could be demonstrated in other trials (Hughes *et al.* 1990; Lonfgren *et al.* 1993; Morris *et al.* 1993).

Diabetes Mellitus

Patients with diabetes mellitus are particularly prone to coronary heart disease, which may be due to atherogenic changes in the lipid profile. Plasma triglycerides are generally decreased and HDL has been inconsistently affected by supplements of fish oils in diabetic patients.

Contradictory findings have been reported in glucose homeostasis in non-insulin dependent diabetes. Some studies have reported improvements (Fasching *et al.* 1991), others no effect (Boberg *et al.* 1992) or deterioration (Vesby & Boberg 1990; Zambon *et al.* 1992). Long-term controlled studies investigating glycaemic control and risk of cardiovascular disease in diabetes are warranted.

Rheumatoid arthritis

Mild to moderate improvements in the symptoms of rheumatoid arthritis have been reported in patients given fish oil supplements (Cleland *et al.* 1988; Kremer *et al.* 1990; Nielsen *et al.* 1992). Fish oil supplements have been found to reduce the need for non-steroidal anti-inflammatory drugs (Belch *et al.* 1988; Skoldstam *et al.* 1992). Supplements of cod liver oil were not found to be of benefit in patients with osteoarthritis (Stammers *et al.* 1992).

Psoriasis

Many studies have demonstrated a mild improvement in psoriasis in patients given fish oil supplements (Bittiner *et al.* 1988; Kojima *et al.* 1991; Maurice *et al.* 1987).

Inflammatory bowel disease

Several clinical trials have evaluated the influence of fish oils in ulcerative colitis. Hawthorn *et al.* (1992) reported mild clinical benefit and reduced requirement for corticosteroids in a double blind controlled trial of fish oil in ulcerative colitis. Similar effects have been reported in other studies (Aslan &

Triadafilopoulus 1992; Lorenz *et al.* 1989; McCall *et al.* 1989; Salomon *et al.* 1990).

Miscellaneous

The effects of fish oils are being investigated in a number of other diseases, including allergic rhinitis, gout, systemic lupus erythematosus (SLE) and multiple sclerosis. Donadio *et al.* (1994) showed that in patients with IgA nephropathy (the most common glomerular disease in the world) treatment with fish oil retarded the rate at which renal function was lost.

More trials are required before fish oils can be recommended for these diseases.

Fish oil is of no proven value in asthma; supplements may lead to deterioration in peak flow rate and an increase in bronchodilator use; deterioration of asthma appears to be more common in aspirin-sensitive patients.

Precautions/contra-indications

Fish oils are best avoided in patients with asthma (particularly those who are aspirin sensitive). Use in diabetes mellitus should be medically supervised with blood glucose monitoring (changes in blood glucose may occur). Use in patients with tendency to haemorrhage or those taking anti-coagulants or anti-platelet drugs should be medically supervised and monitored.

However, patients with asthma, diabetes or those taking anti-coagulants need not be advised to avoid oily fish in the diet.

Pregnancy and breast-feeding

Use in pregnancy should be medically supervised (because of the potential for vitamin A toxicity with excessive intakes of fish liver oil).

Adverse effects

Vitamin A and D toxicity (fish liver oil only). The unpleasant taste of fish liver oil liquids may be masked by mixing with fruit juice or milk.

Interactions

Drugs

Anti-coagulants: may increase the risk of bleeding; use of fish oils should be medically supervised.
Aspirin: may increase the risk of bleeding; use of fish oils in patients on long-term treatment with aspirin should be medically supervised.
Dipyridamole: may increase the risk of bleeding; use of fish oils should be medically supervised.

Nutrients

Vitamin E: fish oils increase the requirement for vitamin E (absolute additional requirements not established, but 3–4 mg vitamin E per gram of total EPA/DHA appears to be adequate; sufficient amounts of vitamin E are added to most fish oil supplements; there is unlikely to be a need for any extra).

Dose

Dietary supplements provide 100–1500 mg combined EPA/DHA per dose; clinical trials of fish oil supplements showing beneficial effects have often used 3–4 g daily (combined EPA/DHA), but these doses should not be used without medical supervision; doses of 1–2 g daily are adequate.

Note: Intake of cod liver oil should not be increased above the doses recommended on the product label to achieve higher intakes of EPA/DHA (risk of vitamin A and D toxicity). Several capsules of cod liver oil could be required to provide the same amount of EPA/DHA as a single dose of cod liver oil liquid. There is no risk of vitamin toxicity with one dose of cod liver oil liquid, but toxicity is likely if several capsules are ingested (vitamin concentration is usually higher in capsules).

Note: fish oil supplements are not identical; they provide different amounts of EPA/DHA. The EPA/DHA content of fish oil supplements is shown in Appendix 1.

References

Anti M., Marra G., Armelao F., Bartoli G.M., Ficarelli R., Percesepe A., de Vitis I., Maria G., Sofo L., Rappacinin G.L., Gentiloni N., Piccioni E. & Miggiano G. (1992) Effect of omega-3 fatty acids on rectal mucosal cell proliferation in subjects at risk for colon cancer. *Gastroenterology* **103**, 883–91.

Aslan A. & Triadafilopoulos G. (1992) Fish oil fatty acid supplementation in active ulcerative colitis: a double-blind, placebo-controlled, crossover study. *American Journal of Gastroenterology* **87**, 432–7.

Belch J.J.F., Ansell D., Madhok R., O'Dowd A. & Sturrock R.D. (1988) Effects of altering dietary fatty acids on requirements for non-steroidal anti-inflammatory drugs in patients with rheumatoid arthritis: a double-blind placebo controlled study. *Annals of Rheumatic Diseases* **47**, 96–104.

Bittiner S.B., Tucker W.F.G., Cartwright I. & Bleehen S.S. (1988) A double-blind, randomized, placebo-controlled trial of fish oil in psoriasis. *Lancet* **i**, 378–80.

Boberg M., Pollare T. & Siegbahn A. (1992) Supplementation with n-3 fatty acids reduces triglycerides but increases PAI-1 in non-insulin dependent diabetes mellitus. *European J of Clinical Investigation* **22**, 645–50.

Bonna K.H., Bjerve K.S. & Straume B. (1990) Effect of eicosapentaenoic and docosahexaenoic acids on blood pressure in hypertension. *New Engl J Med* **322**, 795–801.

Burr M.L., Fehily A.M. & Gilbert J.F. (1989) Effects of changes in fat, fish and fibre intakes on death and myocardial infarction: diet and reinfarction trial (DART). *Lancet* **2**, 757–61.

Cave W.T. (1991) Omega-3 fatty acid diet on tumorigenesis in experimental animals. *World Review of Nutrition & Dietetics* **66**, 462–76.

Chin J.P.F., Gust A.P. & Nestel P.J. (1993) Marine oil dose dependently inhibits vasoconstriction of forearm resistance vessels in humans. *Hypertension* **21**, 22–8.

Christensen J.H., Gustenhoff P. & Ejlersen E. (1993) The effect of n-3 polyunsaturated fatty acids on cardiac ventricular arrhythmias – a pilot study. In: *n-3 fatty acids and vascular disease*, (eds De Caterina et al.) pp 151–7. Springer-Verlag, Berlin.

Cleland L.G., French J.K., Betts W.H., Murphy G.A. & Elliot M.J. (1988) Clinical and biochemical effects of dietary fish oil supplements in rheumatoid arthritis. *Journal of Rheumatology* **15**, 1471–5.

Donadio J.V., Bergstralh E.J., Offord K.P., Spencer D.C. & Holley K.E. (1994) A controlled trial of fish oil in IgA nephropathy. *New Engl J Med* **331**, 1194–9.

Endres S., Ghorbani R. & Kelley V.E. (1989) The effect of dietary supplementation with n-3 polyunsaturated fatty acids on the synthesis of interleukin-1 and tumour necrosis factor by mononuclear cells. *New England Journal of Medicine* **320**, 265–71.

Fasching P., Ratheiser K. & Waldhausal W. (1991) Metabolic effects of fish oil supplementation in patients with impaired glucose tolerance. *Diabetes* **40**, 583–9.

Fumeron F., Brigant L., Ollivier V., Prost D.D., Driss F., Darcet P., Bard J., Parra H., Fruchart J. & Apfelbaum N. (1991) n-3 polyunsaturated fatty acids raise low-density lipoproteins, high density lipoprotein 2, and plasminogen-activating factor inhibitor in healthy young men. *Am J Clin Nutr* **54**, 118–22.

Hardarson T., Kristinsson A. & Skulladottir G. (1989) Cod liver oil does not reduce ventricular extrasystoles after myocardial infarction. *Journal of Internal Medicine* **226**, 33–7.

Harris W.S. (1989) Fish oils and plasma lipid and lipoprotein metabolism in humans: a critical review. *J Lipid Research* **30**, 785–807.

Hawthorne A.B., Daneshmend T.K., Hawkey C.J., Belluzzi A., Everitt S.J., Holmes G.K., Malkinson C., Shaheen M.Z. & Willars J.E. (1992) Treatment of ulcerative colitis with fish oil supplementation: a prospective 12 month randomised controlled trial. *Gut* **33**, 922–8.

Holroyde C.P., Skutches C.L. & Reichard G.A. (1988) Effect of dietary enrichment with n-3 polyunsaturated fatty acid (PUFA) in metastatic breast cancer. *Proceedings of the Society of Experimental Oncology* **7**, 42.

Hughes G.S., Ringer T.V. & Watts K.C. (1990) Fish oil produces an atherogenic lipid profile in hypertensive men. *Atherosclerosis* **84**, 229–37.

Kenny D., Warltier D.C. & Pleuss J.A. (1992) Effect of omega-3 fatty acids on the vascular response to angiotensin in normotensive men. *American Journal of Cardiology* **70**, 1347–52.

Kestin P., Clifton P., Belling G.B. & Nestle P.J. (1990) n-3 fatty acids of marine origin lower systolic blood pressure and triglycerides but raise LDL cholesterol compared with n-3 and n-6 fatty acids from plants. *Am J Clin Nutr* **51**, 1028–34.

Kojima T., Terano T., Tanabe E., Okamato S., Tamura Y. & Yoshida S. (1991) Long-term administration of highly purified eicosapentaenoic acid provides improvement of psoriasis. *Dermatologica* **182**, 225–30.

Kremer J.M., Lawrence D.A., Jubiz W., DiGiacomo R., Rynes R., Bartholomew L.E. & Sherman M. (1990) Dietary fish oil and olive oil supplementation in patients with rheumatoid arthritis. Clinical and immunological effects. *Arthritis and Rheumatism* **33**, 810–20.

Kristensen S.D., Schmidt E.B. & Andersen H.R. (1987) Fish oil in angina pectoris. *Atherosclerosis* **64**, 13–19.

Lofgren R.P., Wilt T.J. & Nichol K.L. (1993) The effect of fish oil supplementation on blood pressure. *Am J Public Health* **83**, 267–9.

Lorenz R., Weber P.C., Szimnau P., Heldwein W., Strasser T. & Loeschke K. (1989) Supplementation with n-3 fatty acids from fish oil in chronic bowel disease – a randomized, placebo-controlled, double-blind cross-over trial. *Journal of Internal Medicine* **225**, 225–32.

Maurice P.D.L., Allen B.R., Barkley A.S.J., Cockbill S.R., Stammers J. & Bather P.C. (1987) The effects of dietary supplementation with fish oil in patients with psoriasis. *Br J Dermatology* **117**, 599–606.

McCall T.B., O'Leary D., Bloomfield J. & O'Morain C.A. (1989) Therapeutic potential of fish oil in the treatment of ulcerative colitis. *Alimentary Pharmacology & Therapeutics* **3**, 415–24.

Mehta J.L., Lopez L.M. & Lawson D. (1988) Dietary supplementation with omega-3 polyunsaturated fatty acids in patients with stable coronary heart disease. *Am J*

Med **84**, 45–52.

Meydani S.N., Lichtenstein A.H. & Colwell S. (1993) Immunologic effects of national cholesterol education panel step-2 diets with and without fish-derived n-3 fatty acid enrichment. *Journal of Clinical Investigation* **92**, 105–13.

Morris M.C., Taylor J.O., Stampfer M.J., Rosner B. & Sacks F.M. (1993) The effect of fish oil on blood pressure in mild hypertensive subjects: a randomized crossover trial. *Am J Clin Nutr* **57**, 59–64.

Neuringer M., Anderson G.J. & Connor W.E. (1988) The essentiality of omega-3 fatty acids for the development and function of the retina and brain. *Annual Reviews in Nutrition* **8**, 517–41.

Nielsen G.L., Faarvang K.L., Thomsen B.S., Teglbjaerg K.L., Jensen L.T., Hansen T.M., Lervang H.H., Schmidt E.B., Dyberg J. & Ernst E (1992) The effects of dietary supplementation with n-3 polyunsaturated fatty acids in patients with rheumatoid arthritis: a randomized, double-blind trial. *European Journal of Clinical Investigation* **22**, 687–91.

Olsen S.F., Sorensen J.D., Seecher N.J., Hedergaard M., Henricksen T.B., Hansen H.S. & Grant A. (1992) Randomised controlled trial of effect of fish-oil supplementation on pregnancy duration. *Lancet* **339**, 1003–7.

Parks J.S., Kaduck-Sawyer J., Bullock B.C. & Rudel L.L. (1990) Effect of dietary fish oil on coronary artery and aortic atherosclerosis in African green monkeys. *Arteriosclerosis* **10**, 1102–12.

Salomon P., Kornbluth A.A. & Janowitz H.D. (1990) Treatment of ulcerative colitis with fish oil n-3 omega fatty acid: an open trial. *Journal of Clinical Gastroenterology* **12**, 157–61.

Sanders T.A.B., Hinds A. & Perreira C.C. (1989) Influence of n-3 fatty acids on blood lipids in normal subjects. *Journal of Internal Medicine* **225**, Suppl 1, 99–104.

Sanders T.A.B. (1993) Marine oils: metabolic effects and role in human nutrition. *Proc Nutr Soc* **52**, 457–72.

Saynor R., Verel D. & Gillott T. (1984) The long term effect of dietary supplementation with fish lipid concentrate on serum lipids, bleeding time, platelets and angina. *Atherosclerosis* **50**, 3–10.

Schmidt E.B., Kristensen S.D. & De Caterina R. (1993) The effects of n-3 fatty acids on plasma lipids and lipoproteins and other cardiovascular risk factors in patients with hyperlipidaemia. *Atherosclerosis* **103**, 107–21.

Skoldstam L., Borjesson O., Kjallman A., Seiving B. & Akesson B. (1992) Effect of six months of fish oil supplementation in stable rheumatoid arthritis. A double-blind controlled study. *Scandinavian Journal of Rheumatology* **21**, 178–85.

Stammers T., Sibbald B. & Freeling P. (1992) Efficacy of cod liver oil as an adjunct to non-steroidal anti-inflammatory drug treatment in the management of osteoarthritis in general practice. *Annals of Rheumatic Diseases* **51**, 128–9.

Terano T., Salmon J.A., Higg G.A. & Moncada S. (1986) Eicosapentaenoic acid as a modulator of inflammation. Effect on prostaglandin and leukotriene synthesis. *Biochemical Pharmacology* **35**, 779–85.

Vanhoutte P.M., Shimokawa H. & Boulanger C. (1991) Fish oil and the platelet-blood wall vessel interaction. *World Review of Nutrition & Dietetics* **66**, 233–44.

Vessby B. & Boberg M. (1990) Dietary supplementation with n-3 fatty acids may impair glucose tolerance in patients with non-insulin dependent diabetes mellitus. *Journal of Internal Medicine* **228**, 165–71.

Zambon S., Friday K.E. & Childs M.T. (1992) Effect of glyburide and omega-3 fatty acid dietary supplements on glucose and lipid metabolism in patients with non-insulin dependent diabetes mellitus. *Am J Clin Nutr* **56**, 447–54.

Chapter 20
Fluoride

Description
Fluoride is a trace element.

Human requirements
There does not appear to be a physiological requirement for fluoride and, in the UK, no Reference Nutrient Intake has been set, but a safe and adequate intake, for infants only, is 0.05 mg/kg daily.

Action
Fluoride has a marked affinity for hard tissues and forms calcium fluorapatite in teeth and bone. It protects against dental caries and may have a role in bone mineralization. It helps remineralization of bone in pathological conditions of demineralization.

Dietary sources
Foods high in fluoride include sea foods and tea. Cereals and milk are poorer sources. An important source of fluoride is fluorinated drinking water. In the UK, tea provides 70% of the total flouride intake; and if the water is fluorinated, consumption of large volumes of tea can result in fluoride intakes of 4–12 mg daily.

Metabolism

Absorption
Oral fluoride is rapidly absorbed by passive transport from the gastro-intestinal tract; some is absorbed from the stomach and some from the small intestine.

Distribution
Fluoride is found principally in bone and teeth.

Elimination
Elimination is mainly in the urine, with small amounts lost in the sweat (especially in warm climates) and the bile.

Deficiency
No essential function has been clearly established; low levels of fluoride in drinking water are associated with dental caries.

Uses

Dental caries
Fluoride is recommended for the prophylaxis of dental caries in infants and children.

Osteoporosis
Sodium fluoride stimulates bone formation and increases bone mass (Braincon & Meunier 1981; Riggs *et al.* 1990), but the incidence of side effects is high and the structure of the bone formed may be abnormal. There is insufficient evidence to justify fluoride as a treatment for osteoporosis.

Precautions/contra-indications
The British Association for Community Dentistry advises that fluoride is unnecessary for infants under 6 months and that fluoride should not be given in areas where the drinking water contains fluoride levels which exceed 700 µg/l.

Adverse effects
Chalky white patches on the surface of the teeth (may occur with recommended doses); yellow-brown staining of teeth, stiffness and aching of bones (with chronic excessive intake). Symptoms of acute overdosage include:

- diarrhoea,
- nausea,
- gastro-intestinal cramp,
- bloody vomit,
- black stools,
- increased watering of mouth and eyes.
- drowsiness,
- weakness,
- faintness,
- shallow breathing,
- tremors, and

Dose
Systemic fluoride supplements should not be prescribed without reference to the fluoride content of the local water supply (information available from the local Water Board).

Table 20.1 Daily doses[1] of fluoride (expressed as fluoride ion) in infants and children

Fluoride content of water	Under 6 months	6 months – 2 years	2–4 years	Over 4 years
< 300 µg	none	250 µg	500 µg	1 mg
300–700 µg	none	none	250 µg	500 µg
> 700 µg	none	none	none	none

1. Recommended by the British Association for the Study of Community Dentistry.

References
Briancon D. & Meunier P.J. (1981) Treatment of osteoporosis with fluoride, calcium and vitamin D. *Orthop Clin North Am* **12**, 629–48.

Riggs B.L., Hodgson S.F., O'Fallon M., Chao E.Y.S., Wahner H.W., Muhs J.M., Cedel S.L. & Melton L.J. (1990) Effect of fluoride treatment on the fracture rate in postmenopausal women with osteoporosis. *New Engl J Med* **322**, 802–9.

Chapter 21
Folic Acid

Description
Folic acid is a water-soluble vitamin of the vitamin B complex.

Nomenclature
Folic acid (pteroyl glutamic acid) is the parent compound for a large number of derivatives collectively known as folates. Folate is the generic term used to describe the compounds that exhibit the biological activity of folic acid; it is the preferred term for the vitamin present in foods which represents a mixture of related compounds (folates).

Human requirements

Dietary Reference Values for Folic Acid (µg/d)

Age	RNI	EAR	LRNI
0–12 months	50	40	30
1–3 years	70	50	35
4–6 years	100	75	50
7–10 years	150	110	75
11–50+ years	200	150	100
Pregnancy[1]	300		
Lactation	260		

1. The Department of Health recommends that all women who are pregnant or planning a pregnancy should take a folic acid supplement (see Dose)
Reproduced and adapted with the permission of the Controller of Her Majesty's Stationery Office.

Intakes
In the UK the average adult diet provides: for men, 322 µg daily; for women, 224 µg.

Action
Folates are involved in a number of single carbon transfer reactions, especially in the synthesis of purines and pyrimidines (and hence the synthesis of DNA), glycine and methionine. They are also involved in some amino acid conversions and the formation and utilization of formate. Deficiency leads to impaired cell division (effects most noticeable in rapidly regenerating tissues).

Dietary sources

Food portion	Folate content (μg)
Breakfast cereals	
1 bowl All-Bran (45 g)	*80*
1 bowl Bran Flakes (45 g)	**110**
1 bowl Corn Flakes (30 g)	*70*
1 bowl Muesli (95 g)	**130**
1 bowl Start (40 g)	**140**
Cereal products	
Bread, brown, 2 slices	*30*
white, 2 slices	25
wholemeal, 2 slices	*30*
fortified, 2 slices	**70**
1 chapati	10
Milk and dairy products	
½ pint milk, whole, semi-skimmed, or skimmed	15
½ pint soya milk	*50*
1 pot yoghurt (150 g)	25
Cheese, average (50 g)	15
Camembert (50 g)	*50*
Meat	
Liver, lambs, cooked (90 g)	**220**
Kidney, lambs, cooked (75 g)	*60*
Vegetables	
Broccoli, boiled (100 g)	*65*
Brussels sprouts, boiled (100 g)	**110**
Cabbage, boiled (100 g)	*30*
Cauliflower, boiled (100 g)	*50*
Kale, boiled (100 g)	*90*
Lettuce (30 g)	20
Peas, boiled (100 g)	*50*
Potatoes, boiled (150 g)	**145**
Spinach, boiled (100 g)	**100**
1 small can baked beans (200 g)	*45*
Chickpeas, cooked (105 g)	**110**
Red kidney beans (105 g)	*90*
Fruit	
1 orange	*45*
1 large glass orange juice	*40*
Half a grapefruit	20
Yeast	
Brewer's Yeast (10 g)	**400**
Marmite, spread on 1 slice bread	*50*

Excellent source (**bold**); good source (*italics*).
Information derived from *The Composition of Foods*, 5th Edition (1991) is reproduced with the permission of The Royal Society of Chemistry and the Controller of Her Majesty's Stationery Office.

Metabolism

Absorption
Absorption of folate takes place mainly in the jejunum.

Distribution
Folate is stored mainly in the liver. Enterohepatic recycling is important for maintaining serum levels.

Elimination
Excretion of folate is largely renal, but folates may also be eliminated in the faeces (mainly as a result of folate synthesis by the gut microflora). Folates are also found in breast milk.

Bioavailability
Folates leach into cooking water and are destroyed by cooking or food processing at high temperatures.

Deficiency
Signs and symptoms include:

- megaloblastic macrocytic anaemia,
- weakness,
- tiredness,
- irritability,
- forgetfulness,
- dyspnoea,
- anorexia,
- diarrhoea,
- weight loss,
- headache,
- syncope,
- palpitations, and
- glossitis.

In babies and young children, growth may be affected.

Uses

Pregnancy and pre-pregnancy
Women are advised to take supplements of folic acid around the time of conception and in the early weeks of pregnancy to help reduce the risk of neural tube defects. The strongest evidence that folic acid helps to prevent recurrence of neural tube defect comes from a randomized controlled trial involving 1817 women who had had an affected pregnancy and were planning to become pregnant again (MRC Vitamin Study Research Group 1991). Women who were given 4 mg folic acid daily from before they conceived until the 12th week of gestation had about 70% fewer affected pregnancies than those who were given no folic acid supplements or who took no other vitamins.

In a similar trial (Czeizel & Dudas 1992) in 4753 women without a history of affected pregnancy, those given multivitamins, including 0.8 mg of folic acid daily, together with minerals and trace elements had nearly 60% fewer affected pregnancies than those given trace elements only.

Cancer

Poor folic acid status has been associated with megaloblastic changes in the uterine cervix (Whitehead *et al.* 1973) but Butterworth *et al.* (1992) showed that folic acid supplements do not alter the course of established cervical cancer. Megaloblastic changes in the intestinal epithelium have also been linked with poor folate status (Bianchi et al 1970) and a case-control study (Freundenheim *et al.* 1991) indicated that folate intake was negatively correlated with risk of rectal cancer.

Lowered plasma and red blood cell folic acid levels have been associated with bronchial metaplasia in smokers (Heimburger *et al.* 1985) and a preliminary trial in smokers with pre-cancerous lesions of the lung indicated that folic acid supplementation may be useful in this type of dysplasia (Heimburger *et al.* 1988). In 99 patients with ulcerative colitis, folic acid supplementation reduced the incidence of neoplasia by 62% (Lashner *et al.* 1989).

Folate deficiency may be a factor in the initiation of pre-cancerous lesions and further follow-up studies are required. There is insufficient evidence to recommend folic acid supplements for the prevention of cancer.

Precautions/contra-indications

Pernicious anaemia – folic acid will correct the haematological abnormalities, but neuropathy may be precipitated. Doses of folic acid > 400 μg daily are not recommended until pernicious anaemia has been ruled out.

Pregnancy/breast-feeding

No problems reported; supplements are required during pregnancy and when planning a pregnancy (see Dose).

Adverse effects

Folic acid is generally considered to be safe even in high doses, but it may lead to convulsions in patients taking anticonvulsants and may precipitate neuropathy in pernicious anaemia. Some gastro-intestinal disturbance and altered sleep patterns have been reported at doses of 15 mg daily. Allergic reactions (shortness of breath, wheezing, fever, erythema, skin rash, itching) have been reported rarely.

Interactions

Drugs

Anticonvulsants: requirements for folic acid may be increased, but concurrent use of folic acid may antagonize the effects of anticonvulsants; an increase in anticonvulsant dose may be necessary in patients who receive supplementary folic acid (monitoring required).

Antibiotics: may interfere with the microbiological assay for serum and erythrocyte folic acid (falsely low results).

Cholestyramine: may reduce the absorption of folic acid; patients on prolonged cholestyramine therapy should take a folic acid supplement one hour before cholestyramine administration.

Methotrexate: acts as a folic acid antagonist; risk significant with high dose and/or prolonged use (folinic acid instead of folic acid should be used).

Oestrogens (including oral contraceptives): may reduce blood levels of folic acid.

Pyrimethamine: acts as a folic acid antagonist; risk significant with high dose and/or prolonged use; folic acid supplements should be given in pregnancy.

Sulphasalazine: may reduce the absorption of folic acid; requirements for folic acid may be increased.

Trimethoprim: acts as a folic acid antagonist; risk significant with high dose and/or prolonged use.

Nutrients

Adequate amounts of all B vitamins are required for optimal functioning; deficiency or excess of one B vitamin may lead to abnormalities in the metabolism of another.

Zinc: may reduce the absorption of zinc.

Dose

Prevention of first occurrence of neural tube defects in women who are planning a pregnancy: oral, 400 µg daily before conception until 12th week of pregnancy.

Prevention of recurrence of neural tube defects: oral, 5 mg daily before conception until 12th week of pregnancy.

For prophylaxis during pregnancy (after 12th week): oral, 200–500 µg daily.

As a dietary supplement: oral, 100–500 µg daily.

References and further reading

Bianci A., Chipman D.W., Dreskin A. & Rosensweig N.S. (1970) Nutritional folic acid deficiency with megaloblastic changes in the small bowel epithelium. *N Engl J Med* **282**, 859–61.

Butterworth C.E., Hatch K.D., Soong S.J., Cole P., Tamura T., Sauberlich H.E., Borst M., Macaluso M. & Baker V. (1992) Oral folic acid supplementation for cervical dysplasia; a clinical intervention trial. *Am J Obs Gynaecol* **166**, 803–9.

Czeizel A.E. & Dudas I. (1992) Prevention of the first occurrence of neural tube defects by periconceptual vitamin supplementation. *New England Journal of Medicine* **327**, 1832–5.

DoH (1992) *Folic Acid and the Prevention of Neural Tube Defects. Report from an Expert Advisory Group.* HMSO, London.

Freundenheim J.L., Graham S., Marshall J.R., Haughey B.P., Cholewinski S. & Wilkinson G. (1991) Folate intake and carcinogenesis of the colon and rectum. *Int J Epidemiol* **20**, 368–74.

Heimburger D.C., Bailey W.C., Alexander C.B., Birch R., Combs B., Soto P., Saxo D., Schnaper H. & Krumdiek C.L. (1985) Bronchial metaplasia in smokers associated with decreased folic acid levels. *Am Rev Respir Dis* **131**, A392.

Heimburger D.C., Alexander C.B., Birch R., Butterworth C.E., Bailey W.C. & Krumdiek C.L. (1988) Improvement in bronchial squamous metaplasia in smokers treated with folate and vitamin B12: report of a preliminary randomized, double-blind intervention trial. *J Am Med Ass* **259**, 1525–30.

Jagerstad M. & Pietrzik K. (1993) Folate. *Int J Vit Nutr Res* **63**, 285–8.

Lambie D.G. & Johnson R.H. (1985) Drugs and Folate Metabolism. *Drugs* **30**, 145–55.

Lashner B.A., Heidenreich P.A., Su G.L., Kane S.V. & Hanauer S.B. (1989) Effect of folate supplementation on the incidence of dysplasia and cancer in chronic ulcerative colitis. *Gastroenterology* **97**, 255–9.

MRC Vitamin Study Research Group (1991) Prevention of neural tube defects: results of the Medical Research Council Vitamin Study. *Lancet* **338**, 131–7.

Whitehead N., Reyner F. & Lindenbaum J. (1973) Megaloblastic changes in the cervical epithelium: an association with oral contraceptive therapy and reversal with folic acid. *J Am Med Ass* **226**, 1421–4.

Chapter 22
Garlic

Description
Garlic is the fresh bulb of *Allium sativum* which is related to the lily family (Liliaceae).

Constituents
The major constituents of garlic include alliin, allicin, diallyl-disulphide and ajoene, but these compounds form only a small proportion of the compounds that have been isolated from crushed, cooked and dried garlic.

Alliin, present in fresh garlic, is converted by the enzyme allinase into allicin when the garlic bulb is crushed. Allicin can be converted (by heat) into diallyldisulphide which in turn is converted into various sulphide-containing substances that cause the typical smell of garlic. Allicin and diallyldisulphide combine to form ajoene.

Uses
Garlic has been cultivated for thousands of years for medicinal purposes, including bites, tumours, wounds, headache, cancer and heart disease, and also as a pungent flavouring agent for cooking.

Evidence for beneficial effects of garlic is accumulating but is, as yet, incomplete. Interpretation of trials is made difficult by the fact that different forms of garlic are used and that active ingredients may be lost in processing (Kleijnen *et al.* 1989). The use of standardized, dried garlic preparations or fresh garlic appears to result in the most beneficial effects. Extracts or oils prepared by using steam distillation or organic solvents or 'odourless' garlic preparations may have little activity (Mansell & Reckless 1991). Any preparation which produces no odour whatsoever, suggesting that release of the biologically active allicin has not occurred, is unlikely to be clinically effective.

In addition, the early trials of garlic in the late 1970s suffered from significant methodological difficulties, including inappropriate methods of randomization, lack of controls and short duration (Silagy & Neil 1994).

Cardiovascular disease
Garlic appears to have beneficial effects on a number of cardiovascular risk factors including:

- serum lipid profiles,
- coagulation,
- vasodilatation (Mansell & Reckless 1991).
- platelet aggregation,
- thrombolysis, and

Recently, attention has also focused on its potential antioxidant effect (Phelps & Harris 1993).

One placebo-controlled study (Bordia 1981) showed that garlic administration over a period of 6–10 months in the form of its essential oil reduced serum total cholesterol by 18% and lowered triglycerides and low density lipoprotein while increasing high density lipoprotein. In a multicentre placebo-controlled, double blind study carried out in Germany (Mader 1990) using standardized dried garlic tablets (800 mg daily) total cholesterol fell by 11%. In other studies (De A Santos & Grunwald 1993; Jain *et al.* 1993; Vorberg & Schneider 1990) a daily dose of 900 mg standardized garlic powder significantly reduced serum cholesterol. In a further study (Rassoul *et al.* 1992) dried garlic tablets led to a four times greater reduction in serum cholesterol than a lipid-lowering diet alone.

Garlic has been reported to reduce fibrinogen levels (Harenberg *et al.* 1988), to enhance fibrinolysis (Chutani & Bordia 1981; Harenberg *et al.* 1988) and to inhibit thrombocyte aggregation (Kiesewetter *et al.* 1991).

Several studies have shown that garlic can normalize elevated blood pressure in animals, but only a limited number of human studies have been carried out. In one controlled study (Auer *et al.* 1990), administration of dried garlic tablets (800 mg daily) was associated with a significant reduction in blood pressure from 171/102 to 152/89 mm Hg in hypertensive patients. Blood pressure was also reduced when 900 mg of standardized dried garlic was given (De A Santos & Grunwald 1993; Vorberg & Schneider 1990).

Cancer

Preliminary data from *in vitro* studies, animal studies and epidemiological studies suggest that garlic may have a protective effect in cancer development and progression. Results of epidemiological case-control studies in China (You *et al.* 1989) and Italy (Buiatti *et al.* 1989) suggest that garlic may reduce the risk of gastric cancer. Epidemiological studies cannot by themselves establish causal relationships and prospective data on this possible effect of garlic on cancer risk are required.

Antimicrobial activity

Garlic is being investigated for antibacterial, antifungal and antiviral activity, but current evidence is too limited to recommend garlic for the prevention of infections.

Precautions/contra-indications

Hypersensitivity to garlic.

Pregnancy and breast-feeding

No problems reported.

Adverse effects

Unpleasant breath odour; indigestion; and occasional reports of hypersensitivity reactions including contact dermatitis and asthma. A spinal haematoma (isolated report) has been attributed to the antiplatelet effects of garlic.

Interactions

None established.

Dose

900 mg daily of a standardized garlic product has been used in several studies.

References

Auer W., Eiber A., Hertkorn E., Hoehfeld E., Koehrle U. & Lorenz A. (1990) Hypertension and hyperlipidaemia: garlic helps in mild cases. *Br J Clin Pract* **44** (suppl 69), 3–6.

Bordia A. (1981) Effect of garlic on blood lipids in patients with coronary heart disease. *American Journal of Clinical Nutrition* **34**, 2100–3.

Buiatti E., Palli D. & Declari A. (1989) A case control study of gastric cancer and diet in Italy. *International Journal of Cancer* **44**, 611–6.

Chutani S.K. & Bordia A. (1981) The effect of fried versus raw garlic on fibrinolytic activity in man. *Atherosclerosis* **38**, 417–21.

De A. Santos O.S. & Grunwald J. (1993) Effect of garlic powder tablets on blood lipids and blood pressure – a six month placebo controlled, double blind study. *Br J Clin Res* **4**, 37–44.

Harenberg J., Giese C. & Zimmerman R. (1988) Effect of dried garlic on blood coagulation, fibrinolysis, platelet aggregation and serum cholesterol levels in patients with hyperlipoproteinaemia. *Atherosclerosis* **74**, 247–9.

Jain A.K., Vargas R., Gotzkowsky S. & McMahon F.G. (1993) Can garlic reduce levels of serum lipids? A controlled clinical study. *Am J Med* **94**, 632–5.

Kiesewetter H., Jung E., Pindur G., Jung E.M., Mrowietz C. & Wenzel E. (1991) Effect of garlic on thrombocyte aggregation, microcirculation and other risk factors. *Int J Clin Pharmacol, Ther Toxicol* **29**, 151–5.

Kleijnen J., Knipschild P. & Ter Riet G. (1989) Garlic, onions and cardiovascular risk factors. A review of the evidence from human experiments with emphasis on commercially available preparations. *Br J Clin Pharmacol* **28**, 533–44.

Mader F.H. (1990) Treatment of hyperlipidaemia with garlic-powder tablets. *Azneim-Forsch/Drug Research* **40**, 3–8.

Mansell P. & Reckless J.P. (1991) Garlic. *Br Med J* **303**, 379–80.

Phelps S. & Harris W.S. (1993) Garlic supplementation reduces the susceptibility to oxidation of apolipoprotein B-containing lipoproteins. *Lipid* **28**, 475–7.

Rassoul F., Richter V. & Rotzsch W. (1992) Total and HDL cholesterol screening in the town of Leipzig. *European Journal of Clinical Research* **3A**, 9.

Silagy S. & Neil A. (1994) Garlic as a lipid lowering agent – a meta-analysis. *Journal of the Royal College of Physicians of London* **28**, 39–45.

Vorberg G. & Schneider B. (1990) Therapy with garlic: results of a placebo-controlled, double-blind study. *Br J Clin Pract* **44** (suppl 69), 7–11.

You W.C., Blot W.J. & Chang Y.S. (1989) Allium vegetables and reduced risk of stomach cancer. *J Natl Cancer Inst* **81**, 162–4.

Chapter 23
Germanium

Description
Germanium is an ultratrace mineral.

Human requirements
There is no evidence that germanium is required in human nutrition.

Intakes
The UK diet appears to provide about 200–500 µg daily.

Action
The functions of germanium have not been established but it may act as an antioxidant.

Dietary sources
Meat, dairy produce, vegetables and unrefined cereals provide similar quantities of germanium. Garlic is a particularly rich source.

Metabolism

Absorption
Germanium is rapidly and almost completely absorbed from the gastro-intestinal tract.

Elimination
Elimination is mainly in the urine.

Deficiency
Not established.

Uses
Germanium has been claimed to be effective in the following conditions:

- cardiovascular disease (angina pectoris, hyperlipidaemia, hypertension, myocardial infarction, stroke and Raynaud's disease);
- arthritis;
- burns;
- cancer; and
- prevention of osteoporosis.

None of these claims has been substantiated. Its use is not recommended (see Adverse effects).

Adverse effects

Germanium supplements have been associated with renal damage (Anonymous 1989; van der Spoel *et al*. 1990). In the UK, the Department of Health has recommended that germanium should not be taken as a dietary supplement. Minor skin eruptions and mild diarrhoea have also been reported.

Dose

Supplements should be avoided.

References

Anonymous (1989) Germanium dangers. *Lancet* **334**, 755.
van der Spoel J.I., Stricker B.H., Esseveld M.R., & Schipper M.E.I. (1990) Dangers of germanium supplements. *Lancet* **336**, 117.

Chapter 24
Ginkgo Biloba

Description
Ginkgo biloba is an extract from the dried leaves of *ginkgo biloba* (maidenhair tree).

Constituents
The leaf contains amino acids, flavonoids, and terpenoids (including bilobalide and ginkgolides A, B, C, J, M).

Action
The pharmacological properties of ginkgo biloba have been reviewed (Braquet 1987; Kleijnen & Knipschild 1992). Ginkgo biloba extract has the following properties. It:

- antagonizes platelet activating factor (PAF), reducing platelet aggregation and decreasing the production of oxygen free radicals (Chung *et al.* 1987; Braquet 1991);
- increases blood flow and reduces blood viscosity (Jung *et al.* 1990);
- has free radical scavenging properties (Pincemail *et al.* 1989; Robak & Gryglewski 1988); and
- may influence neurotransmitter metabolism (Defeudis 1991).

Uses

Cerebral insufficiency
The main interest in ginkgo has focused on its use in cerebral insufficiency and it is licensed for this indication in Germany. Over 40 controlled trials have been published (Kleijnen & Knipschild 1992). All trials but one showed positive effects of ginkgo compared with placebo in cerebral insufficiency, which may include symptoms such as:

- difficulties of concentration,
- poor memory,
- confusion,
- absent mindedness,
- lack of energy,
- reduced physical performance,
- tiredness,
- depressed mood,
- anxiety,
- dizziness,
- headache and,
- tinnitus.

However, ginkgo is not effective for such symptoms if they are not associated with cerebral insufficiency.

Miscellaneous
Ginkgo biloba has also been investigated for the treatment of intermittent

claudication and Raynaud's syndrome, and in post-stroke management. Many of the trials carried out are flawed in design. However one of the best trials (Bauer 1984) showed an increase in walking distance with ginkgo compared with placebo.

Ginkgo biloba is currently being investigated for asthma and for other conditions where there are high levels of platelet activating factor, such as burns and inflammatory skin diseases.

Other claims for the value of ginkgo biloba include:

- treatment of Alzheimer's disease, dizziness, haemorrhoids, impotence, macular degeneration of the eye, migraine, tinnitus;
- preventing organ rejection after transplant surgery; and
- reducing blood pressure.

There is no good scientific evidence to support these claims. (Ginkgo biloba is of use in dizziness and tinnitus only when associated with cerebral insufficiency.)

Precautions/contra-indications
Ginkgo biloba should not be used for the treatment of disease without medical supervision. It is contra-indicated in hypotension.

Pregnancy and breast-feeding
Contra-indicated in pregnancy.

Adverse effects
There are few reports of serious toxicity. Headache, nausea, vomiting, heartburn, and diarrhoea have been reported occasionally. There have been rare reports of severe allergic reactions including skin reactions (e.g. itching, erythema and blisters) and convulsions.

Dose
Most clinical trials have used doses of 80–120 mg (occasionally 160–240 mg) daily.

References and further reading
Anonymous (1986) Extract of Ginkgo biloba (EGb 761). *Presse Med* **15**, 1438–1598.

Bauer U. (1984) 6 month double-blind randomised trial of Ginkgo biloba extract versus placebo in two parallel groups in patients suffering from peripheral arterial insufficiency. *Arzneimittelforschung* **34**, 716–20.

Braquet P. (1987) The ginkgolides: platelet activating factor antagonists isolated from Ginkgo biloba: Chemistry, pharmacology and clinical applications. *Drugs of the Future* **12**, 643–99.

Braquet P. & Hosford D. (1991) Ethnopharmacology and the development of natural PAF antagonists as therapeutic agents. *J Ethnopharmacol* **32**, 135–9.

Chung K.F., Dent G., McCusker M., Guinot P.H., Page C.P. & Barnes P.J. (1987) Effect of a ginkgolide mixture (BN 52063) in antagonising skin and platelet responses to platelet activating factor in man. *Lancet* i, 248–51.

Defeudis F.G. (1991) Ginkgo biloba extract (EGb 761): pharmacological activities and clinical applications. *Editions Scientifiques*, Elsevier, Paris pp 78–84.

Jung F., Mrowietz C., Kiesewetter H. & Wenzel E. (1990) Effect of ginkgo biloba on fluidity of blood and peripheral microcirculation in volunteers. *Arznei-mittelforschung* **40**, 589–93.

Kleijnen J. & Knipschild P. (1992) Ginkgo biloba for cerebral insufficiency. *Br J Clin Pharmacol* **34**, 352–58.

Pincemail J., Dupuis M. & Nasr C. (1989) Superoxide anion scavenging effect and superoxide dismutase activity of Ginkgo biloba extract. *Experientia* **45**, 708–12.

Robak J. & Gryglewski R.J. (1988) Flavonoids are scavengers of superoxide anions. *Biochem Pharmacol* **37**, 837–41.

Chapter 25
Ginseng

Description

Ginseng is the dried root of Panax ginseng. There are eight species of genus Panax which are grown in the central Himalayas, China, Korea, Japan and North America. The eight species of Panax are:

- ginseng,
- japonicus,
- notoginseng,
- pseudoginseng,

- quinquefolium,
- stipuleantus
- trifolus, and
- zingigerensis.

Siberian, Manchurian and Brazilian ginseng are commonly referred to as 'ginseng' but do not belong to the genus Panax. The botanical name for Siberian ginseng is *Eleutherococcus senticocus* and for Brazilian ginseng, *Pfaffia paniculata*.

The use of precise terminology is important because the action of the different 'ginsengs' varies. Some dietary supplements do not contain ginsenosides (Cui *et al.* 1994) because they do not contain Panax ginseng.

Constituents

Panax ginseng contains complex mixtures of saponins known as ginsenosides or panaxosides; at least 20 saponins have been isolated from ginseng roots. However, species vary in composition and concentration.

Eleutherococcus senticocus contains the saponins known as eleutherosides. Neither *Eleutherococcus senticocus* nor *Pfaffia paniculata* contain ginsenosides.

Action

Ginseng has a wide range of pharmacological effects, but their clinical significance in humans has not been fully investigated. Differences in composition of the different species lead to differences in activity.

Analgesic activity, anti-pyretic activity, anti-inflammatory activity, CNS-stimulating and CNS-depressant activity, hypotensive and hypertensive activity, histamine-like activity and antihistamine activity, hypoglycaemic activity and erythropoietic activity have been reported (Hikino 1991). Opposing activities such as hypertension and hypotension are thought to be a result of different ginsenosides in one preparation.

The most consistent biochemical explanation for the effects of the ginsenosides is a facilitating influence on the hypothalamic–pituitary–adrenal axis (Filaretov *et al.* 1988; Fulder 1981). Interactions with central cholinergic (Benishin *et al.* 1991) and dopaminergic mechanisms (Watanabe *et al.* 1991) have also been demonstrated.

Uses

Ginseng is an ancient remedy which has been used for thousands of years in the East. A number of extravagant claims have been made for it, including aphrodisiac and anti-ageing properties. It is not claimed to cure any specific disease, but to restore general vitality.

Ginseng is claimed to be useful for:

- improving stamina;
- alleviating symptoms of tiredness and exhaustion;
- headaches;
- amnesia and mental function;
- improving libido and sexual vigour and preventing impotence;
- regulating blood pressure;
- preventing diabetes mellitus;
- preventing signs of old age and extending youth;
- improving immunity; and
- reducing the risk of cancer.

Available evidence for some of these claims has come mainly from animal studies including:

- increased adaptability to stress (Bittles *et al*. 1979);
- increasing stamina (Brekhman & Dardymov 1969);
- decreasing learning time (Saito *et al*. 1977);
- reduction in blood pressure (Lee *et al*. 1981);
- anti-inflammatory activity (Yuan *et al*. 1983); and
- improved sleep (Lee *et al*. 1990).

In humans ginseng has been shown to increase stamina in athletes (Brekhman 1957) and concentration in radio operators (Medvedev 1963).

Precautions/contra-indications

Ginseng should be avoided by patients with cardiovascular disease (including hypertension), diabetes mellitus, asthma, schizophrenia and other disorders of the nervous system.

Pregnancy and breast-feeding

Avoid.

Adverse effects

Ginseng is relatively non-toxic, but in high doses (> 3 g daily) the following symptoms may occur:

- insomnia;
- nervous excitation;
- euphoria;
- nausea and diarrhoea (especially in the morning);
- skin eruptions;
- oedema;
- oestrogenic effects (e.g. breast tenderness and temporary return of menstruation in post-menopausal women).

Interactions

Drugs

Tranquillisers: ginseng may reverse the effects of sedatives and tranquillisers.

Dose

Not established.

References and further reading

Benishin C.G., Lee R., Wang L.C.H. & Liu H.J. (1991) Effects of ginsenoside Rb-1 on central cholinergic metabolism. *Pharmacology* **42**, 223–9.

Bittles A.H., Fulder S.J., Grant E.C. & Nicholls W. (1979) The effect of ginseng on lifespan and stress response in mice. *Gerontology* **25**, 125–31.

Brekhman I.I. (1957) *Zenschen*. Medgiz, Leningrad.

Brekhman I.I. & Dardymov I.V. (1969) New substances of plant origin which increase adaptation to non-specific stress. *Ann Rev Pharmacol* **9**, 419–30.

Cui J., Garle M., Eneroth P. & Bjorkhem (1994) What do commercial ginseng preparations contain? *Lancet* **344**, 134.

Filaretov A.A., Bogdanova T.S., Podvigina T.T. & Bogdanov A.L. (1988) Role of pituitary–adrenocortical system in body adaptation possibilities. *Exp Clin Endocrinol* **92**, 129–36.

Fulder S. (1981) Ginseng and the hypothalamic control of stress. *Am J Chinese Med* **9**, 112–8.

Hikino, H. (1991) Traditional remedies and modern assessment: the case of ginseng. In Wijesekera R.O.B. (ed.) *The Medicinal Plant Industry*, CRC Press, Boca Raton, Florida.

Hiroshi H. (1991) Traditional Remedies and Modern Assessment: The Case of Ginseng. In: *The Medicinal Plant Industry* (ed. R.O.B. Wijesekera), p 151. CRC Press, London.

Lee D.C., Lee M.O., Kim C.Y. & Clifford D.H. (1981) Effect of ether, ethanol, and aqueous extracts of ginseng on cardiovascular function in dogs. *Can J Comp Med* **45**, 182–5.

Lee S.P., Honda K., Ho-Rhee Y. & Inoue S. (1990) Chronic intake of Panax ginseng extract stabilises sleep and wakefulness in sleep-deprived rats. *Neuroscience Letter* **111**, 217–21.

Medvedev M.A. (1963) The effect of ginseng on the working performance of radio operators. In: *Papers on the Study of Ginseng and Other Medicinal Plants of the Far East*, **Vol 5**. Primorskoe Knizhnoe Izdatelsvo, Vladivostok.

Saito H., Tschuiya M., Naka S. & Takugi K. (1977) Effects of Panax Ginseng root on conditioned avoidance response in rats. *Jpn J Pharmacol* **27**, 509–16.

Watanebe H., Ohta-Himamura L., Asakura W., Matoba Y. & Matsumota K. (1991) Effect of Panax ginseng on age-related changes in the spontaneous motor activity and dopaminergic system in rat. *Jpn J Pharmacol* **55**, 51–6.

Yuan W.X., Gui L.H., Zhou J.Y., Li Q.Y. & Yu Q.H. (1983) Some pharmacological effects of ginseng saponins. *Zhongguo Yaoli Zuebo* **4**, 124–8.

Chapter 26
Green-lipped mussel

Description

Green-lipped mussel is an extract of the green-lipped mussel (*Perna canaliculata*), which is a salt-water shellfish, indigenous to New Zealand.

Constituents

Green-lipped mussel contains a weak anti-inflammatory agent and also amino acids, fats, carbohydrates and minerals.

Uses

Green-lipped mussel is claimed to be effective in the treatment of rheumatoid arthritis. The small number of human studies published have generally shown that green-lipped mussel is not effective in arthritis (Caughey *et al.* 1983; Huskisson *et al.* 1981; Larkin *et al.* 1985), but two studies have shown positive effects (Gibson & Gibson 1981; Gibson *et al.* 1980). Evidence to show that green-lipped mussel works is equivocal.

Adverse effects

Green-lipped mussel is relatively non-toxic, but allergic reactions (e.g. gastro-intestinal discomfort, nausea and flatulence) have been reported occasionally.

Dose

Not established; dietary supplements provide approximately 1 g per daily dose.

References

Caughey D.E., Grigor R.R. & Caughey E.B. (1983) Perna canaliculus in the treatment of rheumatoid arthritis. *Eur J Rheumatol Inflamm* **6**, 197–200.

Gibson R.G., Gibson S.L., Conway V. & Chapell D. (1980) Perna canaliculus in the treatment of arthritis. *Practitioner* **224**, 955–60.

Gibson R.G. & Gibson S.L. (1981) Seatone in arthritis. *Br Med J* **282**, 1795.

Huskisson E.C., Scott J. & Bryans R. (1981) Seatone is ineffective in arthritis. *Br Med J* **282**, 1358–9.

Larkin J.G., Capell H.A. & Sturrock R.D. (1985) Seatone in rheumatoid arthritis: a six-month placebo-controlled study. *Ann Rheum Dis* **44**, 199–201.

Chapter 27
Guarana

Description
Guarana is produced from the seeds of a South American shrub, *Paullinia Cupana*, which are dried and powdered.

Constituents
It contains a substance named guaranine (a synonym for caffeine).

Action
Guarana, like coffee, acts as a CNS stimulant.

Uses
Guarana is claimed to:

- improve mental alertness, endurance, vitality, immunity, stamina in athletes and sexual drive;
- retard aging;
- alleviate migraine, diarrhoea, constipation and tension; and
- act as an appetite suppressant to aid slimming;

but it has not been subject to controlled trials.

Precautions/contra-indications
Guarana is best avoided at bedtime.

Pregnancy and breast-feeding
Avoid.

Adverse effects
Guarana may cause:

- insomnia,
- nervousness,
- irritability,
- palpitations,
- flushing, and
- elevated blood pressure.

Chapter 28
Inositol

Description
Inositol is associated with the B Complex, but is not an officially recognized vitamin. It is an active constituent of dietary lecithin. There are 9 isomers of inositol. (Myoinositol is the most abundant and biologically active.)

Human requirements
No proof exists for a dietary need by humans. It appears that the average intake from foods is adequate for health.

Intakes
The UK diet appears to provide approximately 1 g of myoinositol daily. Inositol can be synthesized in several tissues (including brain, kidney, liver, mammary gland and testis) from D-glucose. Approximately 4 g of inositol per day can be synthesized in the human kidney.

Action
Inositol functions as a phospholipid component of membranes and lipoproteins and modulates the activity of several membrane-bound enzymes. It maintains the selective permeability of plasma membranes and serves as a source of releasable arachidonic acid for eicosanoid synthesis. It is important for early growth and development. Myoinositol is also involved in the mobilization of intracellular calcium.

Dietary sources
Good sources of inositol include heart, liver, beans, wholegrains, nuts, cantaloupe melons and citrus fruits. Inositol is added to infant milk formulae.

Metabolism

Absorption
Absorption occurs in the small intestine by active transport.

Elimination
Inositol is eliminated primarily in the urine. The kidney plays a crucial part in the regulation of inositol status and, in renal failure, inositol levels increase (Holub 1984). These high circulating levels of inositol could have neurotoxic effects.

Deficiency
No specific symptoms of inositol deficiency have been reported in humans.

Uses

Inositol is claimed to be useful in the treatment of diabetes. The myoinositol content of the nerves of diabetic patients is reduced and oral supplementation improves nerve function in some diabetic patients (Holub 1984, 1986), but there is currently no justification for recommending inositol as a dietary supplement to diabetic patients.

Claims that inositol acts as a lipid-lowering agent need further investigation. Therapeutic administration of myoinositol has resulted in small reductions in plasma cholesterol levels in some hypercholesterolaemic patients, but minor elevations in others (Select Committee on GRAS substances 1975).

Clinical interest in inositol has focused in its role in growth and development. Hallman *et al.* (1992) reported that inositol supplements increased survival in premature infants with respiratory distress syndrome.

Despite claims to the contrary, inositol has not been a successful treatment for alopecia and tone deafness.

Adverse effects

None reported except mild diarrhoea.

Dose

None established. Dietary supplements provide 250–750 mg per dose.

References

Hallman M., Bry K., Hoppu K., Lappi M. & Pohjavuori M. (1992) Inositol supplementation in infants with respiratory distress syndrome. *New Engl J Med* **326**, 1233–9.

Holub B.J. (1984) Nutritional, biochemical and clinical aspects of inositol and phosphatidylinositol metabolism. *Can J Physiol Pharmacol* **62**, 1–8.

Holub B. (1986) Metabolism and function of myo-inositol and inositol phospholipids. *Ann Rev Nutr* **6**, 563–97.

Select Committee on GRAS substances (1975) *Evaluation of the health aspects of inositol as a food ingredient*. NTIS PB262660.

Chapter 29
Iodine

Description
Iodine is an essential trace element.

Human requirements

Dietary Reference Values for Iodine (µg/d)

Age	RNI	LRNI
0–3 months	50	40
4–12 months	60	40
1–3 years	70	40
4–6 years	100	50
7–10 years	110	55
11–14 years	130	65
15–50+ years	140	70
Pregnancy	140	70
Lactation	140	70

Note: No EAR has been derived for iodine.
Reproduced and adapted with the permission of the Controller of Her Majesty's Stationery Office.

Intakes
In the UK the average adult diet provides: for men, 251 mcg daily; for women, 184 µg.

Action
Iodine is an essential part of the thyroid hormones, thyroxine (T_4) and triiodothyronine (T_3).

Dietary sources

Food portion	Iodine content (µg)
Milk and dairy products	
½ *pint milk, whole, semi-skimmed or skimmed*	45
1 *pot yoghurt (150 g)*	90
Cheese (50 g)	25
Fish	
Cod, cooked (150 g)	**150**
Haddock, cooked (150 g)	**300**
Mackerel, cooked (150 g)	**200**
Plaice, cooked (150 g)	50

Excellent sources (**bold**); good sources (*italics*).
Note: Iodized salt contains 150 µg/5 g.
Information derived from *The Composition of Foods*, 5th Edition (1991) is reproduced with the permission of The Royal Society of Chemistry and the Controller of Her Majesty's Stationery Office.

Metabolism

Absorption
Inorganic iodine is rapidly and efficiently absorbed. Organically bound iodine is less well absorbed.

Distribution
Iodine is transported to the thyroid gland (for the synthesis of thyroid hormones), and to a lesser extent to the salivary and gastric glands.

Elimination
Excretion of inorganic iodine is mainly in the urine. Some organic iodine is eliminated in the faeces. Iodine is excreted in the breast milk.

Deficiency
Iodine deficiency leads to goitre and hypothyroidism.

Uses
Supplements containing iodine may be required by vegans (strict vegetarians who consume no dairy products). In a study in Greater London which included 38 vegans (Draper *et al*. 1993) intakes of iodine in the vegan individuals were below the dietary reference values. The authors of the study concluded that the impact of these low iodine intakes should be studied further and that vegans should use appropriate dietary supplements.

Pregnancy and breast-feeding
Doses exceeding the Reference Nutrient Intake should not be used (may result in abnormal thyroid function in the infant).

Adverse effects
High iodine intake may induce hyperthyroidism (particularly in those over the age of 40 years) and toxic modular goitre or hypothyroidism in patients

with autoimmune thyroid disease. There is a risk of hyperkalaemia with prolonged use of high doses. Toxicity is rare with intakes below 5000 µg daily and extremely rare at intakes below 1000 µg daily.

Hypersensitivity reactions including, headache, rashes, symptoms of head cold, swelling of lips, throat and tongue, and arthralgia (joint pain) have been reported.

Interactions

Drugs
Antithyroid drugs: iodine may interfere with thyroid control.

Interference with diagnostic tests
Iodine administration may interfere with thyroid function tests.

Dose
As a dietary supplement, a dose of 1000 µg daily should not be exceeded.

References
Draper A., Lewis J., Malhotra N., Wheeler E. (1993) The energy and nutrient intakes of different types of vegetarian: a case for supplements? *Br J Nutr* **69**, 3–19.

Chapter 30
Iron

Description
Iron is an essential trace mineral.

Human requirements

Dietary Reference Values for Iron (mg/d)

Age	RNI	EAR	LRNI
0–3 months	1.7	1.3	0.9
4–6 months	4.3	3.3	2.3
7–12 months	7.8	6.0	4.2
1–3 years	6.9	5.3	3.7
4–6 years	6.1	4.7	3.3
7–10 years	8.7	6.7	4.7
Males			
11–18 years	11.3	8.7	6.1
19–50+ years	8.7	6.7	4.7
Females			
11–50 years	14.8	11.4	8.0
50+ years	8.7	6.7	4.7
Pregnancy	14.8	11.4	8.0
Lactation	14.8	11.4	8.0

Reproduced and adapted with the permission of the Controller of Her Majesty's Stationery Office.

Intakes
In the UK the average adult diet provides: for men 14.5 mg daily; for women, 12.9 mg. Dietary iron consists of haeme and non-haeme iron; in animal foods about 40% of the iron is haeme iron and 60% is non-haeme iron; all the iron in vegetable products is non-haeme iron.

Action
Iron is a component of haemoglobin, myoglobin and many enzymes which are involved in a variety of metabolic functions, including

- transport and storage of oxygen,
- the electron transport chain,
- DNA synthesis, and
- catecholamine metabolism.

Dietary sources

Food portion	Iron content (mg)
Breakfast cereals	
1 bowl All-Bran (45 g)	5
1 bowl Bran Flakes (45 g)	9
1 bowl Corn Flakes (30 g)	2
1 bowl Muesli (95 g)	5
2 pieces Shredded Wheat	2
1 bowl Special K (35 g)	4
1 bowl Start (30 g)	5
1 bowl Sultana Bran (35 g)	5
2 Weetabix	3
Cereal products	
Bread, brown, 2 slices	*1.5*
white[1], 2 slices	*1*
wholemeal 2 slices	*2*
1 chapati	*1.5*
1 naan	*3.5*
Pasta, brown, boiled (150 g)	*2.0*
white, boiled (150 g)	*1.0*
Rice, brown, boiled (165 g)	*0.7*
white, boiled (165 g)	*0.3*
Dairy products	
1 egg, size 2 (60 g)	*1*
Meat	
Red meat, roast (85 g)	*2.5*
1 beef steak (155 g)	**5.4**
Minced beef, lean, stewed (100 g)	**3**
1 chicken leg (190 g)	*1*
Liver, lambs, cooked (90 g)	**9**
Kidney, lambs, cooked (75 g)	**9**
Fish	
Cockles (80 g)	**21**
Mussels (80 g)	**6**
Pilchards, canned (105 g)	*2.8*
Sardines, canned (70 g)	*3*
Vegetables	
Green vegetables, average, boiled (100 g)	*1.5*
Potatoes, boiled (150 g)	*0.5*
1 small can baked beans (200 g)	*3*
Lentils, kidney beans or other pulses (105 g)	*2*
Dahl, chickpea (155 g)	**5**
lentil (155 g)	*2.5*
Soya beans, cooked (100 g)	*3*
Fruit	
8 dried apricots	*2*
4 figs	*2.5*
½ an avocado pear	*1.5*
Blackberries (100 g)	1
Blackcurrants (100 g)	1

Food portion	Iron content (mg)
Nuts and chocolate	
20 almonds	1
10 Brazil nuts	1
1 small bag peanuts (25 g)	0.5
Milk chocolate (100 g)	*1.6*
Plain chocolate (100 g)	*2.4*

1. White bread is supplemented with additional iron in the UK.
Excellent sources (**bold**); good sources (*italics*).
Information derived from *The Composition of Foods*, 5th Edition (1991) is reproduced with the permission of The Royal Society of Chemistry and the Controller of Her Majesty's Stationery Office.

Metabolism

Absorption

Absorption of iron occurs principally in the duodenum and proximal jejunum. Absorption of food iron varies between 5% and 15%. Haeme iron is more efficiently absorbed than non-haeme iron. Body iron content is regulated mainly through changes in absorption.

Distribution

Iron is transported in the blood bound to the protein, transferrin, and is stored in the liver, spleen and bone marrow as ferritin and haemosiderin.

Elimination

The body has a limited capacity to eliminate iron and iron can accumulate in the body to toxic amounts. Small amounts are excreted in the faeces, urine, skin, sweat, hair, nails and menstrual blood.

Bioavailability

The absorption of non-haeme iron is enhanced by concurrent ingestion of meat, poultry and fish, and by various organic acids, especially ascorbic acid; it is inhibited by phytates (found in bran and high-fibre cereals), tannins (found in tea and coffee), egg yolk and by some drugs and nutrients (see Interactions). Ferrous salts are more efficiently absorbed than ferric salts.

Deficiency

Iron deficiency leads to microcytic hypochromic anaemia. Symptoms include fatigue, weakness, pallor, dyspnoea on exertion and palpitations. Non-haematological effects include impairment in work capacity, intellectual performance, neurological function and immune function, and, in children, behavioural disturbances. Gastro-intestinal symptoms are also fairly common and the fingernails may become lustreless, brittle, flattened and spoon-shaped.

Uses

Requirements may be increased and/or supplements needed in:

- infants and children from the age of 6 months to 4 years;

- early adolescence;
- females during the reproductive period;
- pregnancy; and
- vegetarians.

Precautions/contra-indications

Iron supplements should be avoided in:

- conditions associated with iron overload (e.g. haemochromatosis, haemosiderosis, thalassaemia); and
- gastro-intestinal disease, particularly inflammatory bowel disease, intestinal stricture, diverticulitis and peptic ulcer.

Pregnancy and breast-feeding

The Reference Nutrient Intake for iron during pregnancy is no greater than for other adult women. Requirements during pregnancy are partly offset by lack of menstruation and partly by increased efficiency of absorption. Routine iron supplementation is not required in pregnancy, but iron status should be monitored (see review – Anonymous 1994).

Adverse effects

Iron supplements may cause gastro-intestinal irritation, nausea and constipation, which may lead to faecal impaction, particularly in the elderly. Patients with inflammatory bowel disease may suffer exacerbation of diarrhoea. Any reduced incidence of side-effects associated with modified-release preparations may be due to the fact that only small amounts of iron are released in the intestine. Liquid iron preparations may stain the teeth.

Interactions

Drugs

Antacids: reduced absorption of iron; give two hours apart.
Bisphosphanates: reduced absorption of bisphosphanates; give two hours apart.
Co-careldopa: reduced plasma levels of carbidopa and levodopa.
Levodopa: absorption of levodopa may be reduced.
Methyldopa: reduced absorption of methyldopa.
Penicillamine: reduced absorption of penicillamine.
4-Quinolones: absorption of ciprofloxacin, norfloxacin and ofloxacin reduced by oral iron; give two hours apart.
Tetracyclines: reduced absorption of iron and vice versa; give two hours apart.
Trientine: reduced absorption of iron; give two hours apart.

Nutrients

Calcium: calcium carbonate or calcium phosphate may reduce absorption of iron; give two hours apart. (Absorption of iron in multiple formulations containing iron and calcium is not significantly altered.)
Copper: large doses of iron may reduce copper status and vice versa.
Manganese: reduced absorption of manganese.

Vitamin E: large doses of iron may increase requirement for vitamin E; vitamin E may impair haematological response to iron in patients with iron-deficiency anaemia.

Zinc: reduced absorption of iron and vice versa.

Interference with diagnostic tests

Oral iron may interfere with the test for occult blood in stools (iron may cause black discolouration of stools which obscures test result).

Dose

Iron is best taken on an empty stomach, but food reduces the possibility of stomach upsets; oral liquid preparations should be well diluted with water or fruit juice and drunk through a straw.

Dietary supplements provide 5–50 mg per dose; maximum daily dose recommended by MAFF (see p. 15) is 4 mg.

Note: doses are given in terms of elemental iron; patients should be advised that iron supplements are not identical and provide different amounts of elemental iron; iron content of various iron salts commonly used in supplements is shown in Table 30.1.

Table 30.1 Iron content of commonly used iron supplements

Iron Salt	Iron (mg/g)	Iron (%)
Ferrous fumarate	330	33
Ferrous gluconate	120	12
Ferrous glycine sulphate	180	18
Ferrous orotate	150	15
Ferrous succinate	350	35
Ferrous sulphate	200	20
Ferrous sulphate, dried	300	30
Iron amino acid chelate	100	10

References and further reading

Anonymous (1994) Routine iron supplements in pregnancy are unnecessary. *Drug Ther Bull* **32**, 30–1.

Campbell N.R.C. & Hasinoff B.B. (1991) Iron supplements: a common cause of drug interactions. *Br J Clin Pharm* **31**, 251–5.

Chapter 31
Kelp

Description
Kelp is a preparation of dried seaweed of various species.

Constituents
Kelp is a source of several minerals and trace elements, especially iodine.

Uses
Kelp is claimed to be a slimming aid. (Some herbal products containing kelp are licensed in the UK for this purpose.)

Precautions/contra-indications
Kelp should be avoided in patients with thyroid disease. Further, it may be contaminated with toxic trace elements (e.g. antimony, arsenic, lead, strontium).

Pregnancy and breast-feeding
Avoid (contaminants – see Precautions).

Adverse effects
Kelp may impair control of hypothyroidism and hyperthyroidism.

Interactions
Antithyroid drugs: the iodine content may interfere with thyroid control.

Chapter 32
Lactobacillus

Description
Lactobacillus is a genus of bacteria (consisting of many species) which has the ability to ferment carbohydrate to produce lactic acid. Lactobacilli are part of the normal flora of the intestine, vagina and mouth. Lactobacillus acidophilus is the predominant species in the intestine and vagina. *Lactobacillus bulgaricus* is the main species used to produce yoghurt.

Dietary sources
Dairy products; bread and cereals; meat and fish products; beer and fermenting wine. Lactobacilli are used in the food industry as a preservative (e.g. in yoghurt, buttermilk and cheese production).

Action
Lactobacilli play an important role in maintaining the pH of the vagina in the range 4.0–4.5 through glycogen fermentation to lactic acid. The level of glycogen in the vagina is controlled by circulating oestrogens and the natural lactobacilli in the vagina are thought to be the best defence against infection. Lactobacilli are also thought to contribute to the prevention of infection in the intestine.

Uses

Diarrhoea
Lactobacillus has been claimed to be useful for treating diarrhoea. Early studies reviewed by Sandine *et al.* (1972) claimed excellent success rates, but few of these studies were controlled. A study using randomly assigned controls (Clements *et al.* 1983) failed to show a protective effect against enterotoxigenic E Coli and diarrhoea.

Vaginal infections
Use of lactobacillus preparations in vaginal infections has yielded mixed results. A randomized trial of 84 patients with bacterial vaginosis (Fredriccson *et al.* 1989) compared lactobacillus with acetic acid jelly, oestrogen cream and metronidazole. Significant clinical cures were found only in the metronidazole-treated group.

Some species may be more effective than others for the treatment of vaginal and intestinal infections, but it is not clear that dietary supplements contain the lactobacilli species claimed. Clinical efficacy may be reduced because of the lack of control of purity, viability and species of bacteria claimed to be present in many lactobacillus preparations.

Miscellaneous

Many additional claims have been made for the benefits of lactobacillus including:

- improvement of lactose intolerance;
- reduction in serum cholesterol; and
- anti-tumour and immunomodulatory effects.

Evidence for these claims is sparse.

Adverse effects

None.

Dose

Not established.

References and further reading

Clements M.L., Levine M.M., Ristaino P.A., Daya V.E. & Hughes T.P. (1983) Exogenous lactobacillus fed to man – their fate and ability to prevent diarrhoeal disease. *Prog Fd Nutr Sci* **7**, 29–37.

Drutz D.J. (1992) Lactobacillus prophylaxis for Candida vaginitis. *Ann Intern Med* **116**, 419–20.

Fredriccson B., Englund K., Weintraub L., Olund A. & Nord C.E. (1989) Bacterial vaginosis is not a simple disorder. *Gynaecol Obstet Invest* **28**, 156–60.

Fuller R. (1991) Probiotics in human medicine. *Gut* **32**, 439–42.

Sandine W.E., Muralidhara K.S., Elliker P.R. & England D.C. (1972) Lactic acid bacteria in food and health: a review with special reference to enteropathogenic Escherichia Coli as well as certain enteric diseases and their treatment with antibiotics and lactobacilli. *J Milk Food Technol* **35**, 691–702.

Chapter 33
Lecithin

Description and nomenclature
Pure lecithin is known as phosphatidylcholine.

Constituents
One teaspoon (3.5 g) lecithin granules provides on average:

- energy 117 kJ (28 kcal),
- phosphatidyl choline 750 mg,
- phosphatidyl inositol 500 mg,
- choline 100 mg,
- inositol 100 mg, and
- phosphorus 110 mg.

Human requirements
Lecithin is not an essential component of the diet. It is synthesized from choline.

Action
Lecithin is a source of choline (see choline, Chapter 13) and inositol (see inositol, Chapter 28). It is an essential component of cell membranes.

Dietary sources
Soya beans, peanuts, liver, meat, eggs.

Metabolism
About 50% of ingested lecithin enters the thoracic duct intact. The rest is degraded to glycerophosphoryl choline in the intestine, and then to choline in the liver. Plasma choline level reflects lecithin intake.

Deficiency
Not established.

Uses
Lecithin is used as a food additive (an emulsifier, E322) in foods such as margarine, mayonnaise and ice-cream.

Lecithin is claimed to be beneficial in the treatment of disease related to impaired cholinergic function (see Chapter 13).

Claims for the value of lecithin in lowering blood pressure and also in hepatitis, gallstones, psoriasis and eczema are unsubstantiated.

Adverse effects

None reported, but see Chapter 13 (although less likely than choline to produce adverse effects).

Dose

Not established. Lecithin supplements provide between 20% and 90% phosphatidylcholine (depends on the product).

Chapter 34
Magnesium

Description
Magnesium is an essential mineral.

Human requirements

Dietary Reference Values (mg/d)

Age	RNI	EAR	LRNI
0–3 months	55	40	30
4–6 months	60	50	40
7–9 months	75	60	45
10–12 months	80	60	45
1–3 years	85	65	50
4–6 years	120	90	70
7–10 years	200	150	115
11–14 years	280	230	180
15–18 years	300	250	190
Males			
19–50+ years	300	250	190
Females			
19–50+ years	270	200	150
Pregnancy	270	200	150
Lactation	320	200	150

Reproduced and adapted with the permission of the Controller of Her Majesty's Stationery Office.

Intakes
In the UK the average diet provides: for males, 336 mg daily; females, 250 mg daily.

Action
Magnesium is an essential co-factor for enzymes requiring ATP. (These are involved in glycolysis, fatty acid oxidation and amino acid metabolism.) It is also required for:

- the synthesis of RNA and replication of DNA;
- neuromuscular transmission; and
- calcium metabolism.

Dietary sources

Food portion	Magnesium content (mg)
Breakfast cereals	
1 bowl All-Bran (45 g)	*90*
1 bowl Bran Flakes (45 g)	*50*
1 bowl Corn Flakes (30 g)	5
1 bowl Muesli (95 g)	*90*
2 pieces Shredded Wheat	*50*
2 Weetabix	*50*
Cereal products	
Bread, brown, 2 slices	40
white, 2 slices	15
wholemeal, 2 slices	*60*
2 chapati	30
Pasta, brown, boiled (150 g)	*60*
white, boiled (150 g)	25
Rice, brown, boiled (165 g)	*60*
white, boiled (165 g)	15
Milk and dairy products	
½ pint milk, whole, semi-skimmed or skimmed	35
1 pot yoghurt (150 g)	30
Cheese (50 g)	12
1 egg, size 2 (60 g)	10
Meat and fish	
Meat, cooked (100 g)	25
Liver, lambs, cooked (90 g)	20
Kidney, lambs, cooked (75 g)	20
White fish, cooked (150 g)	30
Pilchards, canned (105 g)	40
Sardines, canned (70 g)	35
Shrimps (80 g)	*49*
Tuna, canned (95 g)	30
Vegetables	
Green vegetables, average, boiled (100 g)	20
Potatoes, boiled (150 g)	20
1 small can baked beans (200 g)	*60*
Lentils, kidney beans or other pulses (105 g)	*50*
Fruit	
1 banana	35
1 orange	20
Nuts	
20 almonds	*50*
10 Brazil nuts	*80*
30 Hazel nuts	*50*
30 peanuts	*70*

Excellent sources (**bold**); good sources (*italics*).
Note: Hard drinking water may contribute significantly to intake.
Information derived from *The Composition of Foods*, 5th Edition (1991) is reproduced with the permission of The Royal Society of Chemistry and the Controller of Her Majesty's Stationery Office.

Metabolism

Absorption
Absorption of magnesium occurs principally in the jejunum and ileum by active carrier mediated processes (partly dependent on vitamin D and parathyroid hormone) and by diffusion.

Distribution
Magnesium is widely distributed in the soft tissues and skeleton.

Elimination
Excretion is largely in the urine (magnesium homeostasis is controlled mainly by the kidneys), with unabsorbed and endogenously secreted magnesium in the faeces. Small amounts are excreted in saliva and breast milk.

Bioavailability
Bioavailability appears to be enhanced by vitamin D, but is decreased by phytates and non-starch polysaccharides (dietary fibre).

Deficiency
Signs and symptoms include:

- hypocalcaemia and hypokalaemia;
- muscle spasm, tremor and tetany;
- personality changes, lethargy and apathy;
- convulsions, delirium and coma;
- anorexia, nausea, vomiting, abdominal pain and paralytic ileus, and
- cardiac arrhythmias, tachycardia and sudden cardiac death.

Uses

Cardiovascular disease
Magnesium deficiency has been associated with cardiovascular disease and some epidemiological data have suggested a reduced mortality from coronary artery disease in populations living in hard water areas compared with those living in soft water areas. Other data, however, have indicated no such association (Elwood *et al*. 1980) and a large cohort study (The Caerphilly and Speedwell Collaborative Group, 1984), in which 2512 older men have been followed for 10 years, also provided no evidence of a protective role for magnesium in coronary heart disease.

There is, as yet, insufficient evidence to argue that the UK population has a significant amount of 'subclinical' magnesium deficiency which contributes to the high prevalence of coronary heart disease.

Marginal magnesium status has been implicated in myocardial infarction, but reduced serum magnesium levels found in some myocardial infarct patients may be a result of the infarction rather than the cause of it. However, one double blind placebo controlled study in patients with acute myocardial infarction showed reduced serum triglyceride concentrations and tendencies toward increased high density lipoprotein concentrations after oral magnesium supplementation (Rasmussen *et al*. 1989).

Controlled studies have suggested that intravenous magnesium given early after suspected myocardial infarction could reduce the frequency of serious arrhythmias and mortality. Magnesium slows conduction through the atrioventricular node and has been shown to reduce clinically significant arrhythmias after acute myocardial infarction (Woods 1991).

In the second Leicester Intravenous Magnesium Intervention Trial (LIMIT-2) (Woods *et al.* 1992), 28-day mortality post-infarction was reduced by 24% in a group of patients given magnesium. The evidence from this trial has been challenged by the results of ISIS-4 (ISIS Collaborative Group, 1993), in which an excess of 4% deaths by 35 days post-infarction (statistically not significant) contrasts with the reduction reported in LIMIT-2.

Magnesium may also protect the myocardium both against ischaemic injury and against reperfusion injury (Woods 1991). Further effects of magnesium which are likely to be cardioprotective include inhibition of platelet function (Adams & Mitchell 1979) and coronary vasodilatation, possibly through inhibition of contraction of smooth muscle and the production of endothelium-derived relaxing factor (EDRF) (Gold *et al.* 1990).

There is some evidence that magnesium reduces blood pressure (Dykner & Wester 1983; Widman *et al.* 1993). A 20 millimole increase in daily magnesium intake resulted in a diastolic blood pressure fall of 3.4 mmHg in a trial in Dutch women (Witteman *et al.* 1994). Geleijnse *et al.* (1994) showed a reduction in blood pressure with a low-sodium, high-potassium, high-magnesium salt in older patients with mild to moderate hypertension and suggested that the increased magnesium intake could have contributed to the fall in blood pressure.

However, Nowson & Morgan (1989) showed that magnesium supplementation did not have an additive hypotensive effect in mild hypertensive subjects on a reduced sodium intake. Another group (Cappuccio *et al.* 1985), using a double-blind randomized crossover design, detected no fall in blood pressure with magnesium supplementation, despite a significant increase in plasma magnesium concentration.

Diabetes mellitus

Loss of magnesium in diabetes mellitus has been known for many years. In elderly patients with low erythrocyte magnesium concentration, chronic magnesium administration (4.5 g daily) improved their insulin secretion and glucose handling (Paolisso *et al.* 1992). Of particular interest was the finding that magnesium supplementation decreased insulin requirement (Sjogren *et al.* 1988). Further studies are needed.

Asthma

Intravenous magnesium has been shown to dilate the airways of asthmatics (Noppen *et al.* 1990; Skobeloff *et al.* 1989). High dietary magnesium was related to higher forced expiratory volume (FEV_1) and reduced airway hyperreactivity and self-reported wheezing in the general population (Britton *et al.* 1994). Low magnesium intake might be involved in the aetiology of asthma and chronic-obstructive airways disease, and further studies are warranted.

Miscellaneous

Magnesium has been claimed to be of value in pre-menstrual syndrome, osteoporosis, dysmenorrhoea, migraine and chronic fatigue syndrome, but there is limited scientific evidence for these claims.

Precautions/contra-indications
Doses exceeding the Reference Nutrient Intake are best avoided in renal failure.

Pregnancy and breast-feeding
No problems reported with normal intakes.

Adverse effects
Toxicity from oral ingestion is unlikely in individuals with normal renal function. Doses of 3–5 g have a cathartic effect.

Interactions

Drugs
Alcohol: excessive alcohol intake increases renal excretion of magnesium.
Loop diuretics: increased excretion of magnesium.
4-quinolones: may reduce absorption of 4-quinolones; give two hours apart.
Tetracyclines: may reduce absorption of tetracyclines; give two hours apart.
Thiazide diuretics: increased excretion of magnesium.

Dose
As a dietary supplement, not established. Dietary supplements provide 100–500 mg per dose.

References

Adams J.H. & Mitchell J.R.A. (1979) The effect of agents which modify platelet behaviour and of magnesium ions on thrombus formation *in vivo. Thrombus and Haemostasis* **42**, 603–10.

Britton J., Pavord I., Richards K., Wisniewski A., Knox A., Lewis S, Tattersfield A. & Weiss S. (1994) Dietary magnesium, lung function, wheezing and airway hyper-reactivity in a random adult population sample. *Lancet* **344**, 357–62.

The Caerphilly and Speedwell Collaborative Group (1984) Caerphilly and Speedwell collaborative heart disease studies. *Journal of Epidemiology and Community Health* **38**, 259–62.

Cappuccio F.P., Markandu N.D., Beynon G.W., Shore A.C., Sampson B. & Mac-Gregor G.A. (1985) Lack of effect of oral magnesium on high blood pressure: a double-blind study. *Br Med J* **291**, 235–8.

Dyckner T. & Wester T.O. (1983) Effect of magnesium on blood pressure. *Br Med J* **286**, 1847–9.

Elwood P.C., Sweetman P.M. & Bealey W.H. (1980) Magnesium and calcium in the myocardium: cause of death and area differences. *Lancet* **ii**, 720–2.

Geleijnse J.M., Witteman J.C.M., Bak A.A.A., den Breeijen J.H. & Grobbee D.E. (1994) Reduction in blood pressure with a low sodium, high potassium, high magnesium salt in older subjects with mild to moderate hypertension. *Br Med J* **309**, 436–40.

Gold M.E., Buga G.M., Wood K.S., Byrns R.E., Chaudhuri G. & Ignarro L.J. (1990) Antagonistic modulatory roles of magnesium and calcium on release of endothelium-derived relaxing factor and smooth muscle tone. *Circulation Research* **66**, 355–66.

ISIS Collaborative Group (1993) ISIS-4: randomised study of intravenous magnesium in over 500 000 patients with suspected acute myocardial infarction. *Circulation* **88**, Suppl 1, 292.

Noppen M., Vanmaele L., Impens M. & Schandevyl W. (1990) Bronchodilating effects of intravenous magnesium sulphate in acute severe bronchial asthma. *Chest* **97**, 373–6.

Nowson C.A. & Morgan T.O. (1989) Magnesium supplementation in mild hypertensive patients on a moderately low sodium diet. *Clinical & Experimental Pharmacology & Physiology* **16**, 299–302.

Paolisso G., Sgambato S., Gambardella A., Pizza G., Tesauro P., Varrichio M. & D'Onofrio F. (1992) Daily magnesium supplements improve glucose handling in elderly subjects. *Am J Clin Nutr* **55**, 1161–7.

Rasmussen H.S., Aurup P., Goldstein K., McNair P., Mortensen P.B., Larsen O.G. & Lawaetz H. (1989) Influence of magnesium substitution therapy on blood lipid composition in patients with ischaemic heart disease. A double-blind, placebo controlled study. *Archives of Internal Medicine* **149**, 1050–3.

Sjogren A., Floren C.H. & Nilsson A. (1988) Oral administration of magnesium hydroxide to subjects with insulin dependent diabetes mellitus. Effects on magnesium and potassium levels and on insulin requirements. *Magnesium* **7**, 117–122.

Skobeloff E.M., Spivey W.H., McNamara R.M. & Greenspon L. (1989) Intravenous magnesium sulphate for the treatment of acute asthma in the emergency department. *J Am Med Ass* **262**, 1210–3.

Widman L., Webster P.O., Stegmayr B.K. & Wirell M. (1993) The dose-dependent reduction in blood pressure through administration of magnesium. *Am J Hypertension* **6**, 41–5.

Witteman J.C.M., Grobbee D.E., Derkx F.H.M., Bouillon R., de Bruijn A.A. & Hofman A. (1994) Reduction of blood pressure with oral magnesium supplementation in women with mild to moderate hypertension. *Am J Clin Nutr* **60**, 129–35.

Woods K.L. (1991) Possible pharmacological actions of magnesium in acute myocardial infarction. *British Journal of Clinical Pharmacology* **32**, 3–10.

Woods K.L., Fletcher S., Roffe C. & Haider Y. (1992) Intravenous magnesium sulphate in suspected acute myocardial infarction: results of the second Leicester Intravenous Magnesium Intervention Trial (LIMIT–2). *Lancet* **339**, 1553–8.

Chapter 35
Manganese

Description
Manganese is an essential trace mineral.

Human requirements
No Reference Nutrient Intake or Estimated Average Requirement has been set for manganese in the UK, but a safe and adequate intake is, for adults, 1.4 mg daily; infants, 10 µg daily.

Intakes
In the UK the average adult diet provides 4.6–5.4 mg daily.

Action

Manganese activates several enzymes, including hydroxylases, kinases, decarboxylases and transferases. It is also a constituent of several metalloenzymes, such as arginase, pyruvate carboxylase, and also superoxide dismutase which protects cells from free radical attack. It may have a role in the regulation of glucose homeostasis and in calcium mobilisation.

Dietary sources

Food portion	Manganese content (mg)
Cereal products	
Bread, brown, 2 slices	**1**
white, 2 slices	0.3
wholemeal, 2 slices	**1.5**
Milk and dairy products	
Milk and cheese	Trace
Meat and fish	
Meat and fish	Trace
Lambs liver, cooked (90 g)	0.4
Vegetables	
1 small can baked beans (200 g)	0.6
Lentils, kidney beans or other pulses (105 g)	**1–1.5**
Green vegetables, average, boiled (100 g)	0.2
Fruit	
1 banana	0.5
Blackberries, stewed (100 g)	**1.5**
Pineapple, canned (150 g)	**1.5**

Food portion	Manganese content (mg)
Nuts	
20 almonds	0.3
10 Brazil nuts	0.4
30 Hazel nuts	**1.0**
30 peanuts	0.7
Tea, 1 cup	0.3

Excellent sources (> 1 mg/portion) (**bold**).
Note: Some other foods (e.g. breakfast cereals) contain significant quantities, but there is no reliable information on the amount.
Information derived from *The Composition of Foods*, 5th edition (1991) is reproduced with the permission of The Royal Society of Chemistry and the Controller of Her Majesty's Stationery Office.

Metabolism

Absorption
Absorption of manganese occurs throughout the length of the small intestine, probably via a saturable carrier mechanism, but absorptive efficiency is believed to be poor.

Distribution
Manganese is transported in the blood bound to plasma proteins. Organs with the highest concentrations include the liver, kidney and pancreas, but 25% of the body pool is found within the skeleton. Homeostasis is maintained by hepato-biliary and intestinal secretion.

Elimination
Manganese is eliminated primarily in the faeces.

Bioavailability
Bioavailability of manganese appears to be enhanced by vitamin C and meat-containing diets, but is decreased by iron and non-starch polysaccharides (dietary fibre). Although tea contains large amounts of manganese, it is essentially unavailable to humans.

Deficiency
Manganese deficiency in individuals consuming mixed diets is very rare. Symptoms thought to be associated with deficiency (which have occurred only on semi-purified diets) include:

- weight loss,
- dermatitis,
- hypocholesterolaemia,
- depressed growth of hair and nails, and
- reddening of black hair.

Uses

Diabetes

Manganese has been claimed to be useful in diabetes mellitus. A relationship between dietary manganese and carbohydrate metabolism in humans was suggested by Rubenstein *et al.* (1962). They described the case of a diabetic patient resistant to insulin therapy who responded to oral manganese with a consistent drop in blood glucose levels. However, there is insufficient evidence to warrant recommendation of manganese supplements to patients with diabetes.

Adverse effects

Manganese is essentially non-toxic when administered orally. Toxic reactions in humans occur only as the result of the chronic inhalation of large amounts of manganese found in mines and some industrial plants. Signs include severe psychiatric abnormalities and neurological disorders similar to Parkinson's disease.

Dose

Not established; dietary supplements provide 5–50 mg per dose.

References

Rubenstein A.H., Levin N.W. & Elliot G.A. (1962) Manganese-induced hypoglycaemia. *Lancet* **2**, 1348–51.

Chapter 36
Molybdenum

Description
Molybdenum is an essential ultratrace mineral.

Human requirements
No Reference Nutrient Intake or Estimated Average Requirement has been set for molybdenum in the UK but a safe and adequate intake is, for adults, 50–400 µg daily; infants, children and adolescents, 0.5–1.5 µg/kg daily.

Intakes
Average adult intakes of molybdenum are 120–140 µg daily (USA figures).

Action
Molybdenum functions as an essential cofactor for several enzymes, including:

- aldehyde oxidase (oxidises and detoxifies various pyrimidines, purines and related compounds which are involved in DNA metabolism);
- xanthine oxidase/dehydrogenase (catalyses the formation of uric acid); and
- sulphite oxidase (involved in sulphite metabolism).

Dietary sources
The richest sources of molybdenum include milk and milk products, dried beans and peas, wholegrain cereals and liver and kidney.

Metabolism

Absorption
Molybdenum is readily absorbed, but the mechanism of absorption is uncertain.

Distribution
It is transported in the blood loosely attached to erythrocytes and binds specifically α_2-macroglobulin. The highest concentrations are found in the liver and kidney.

Elimination
Excretion of manganese is mainly via the kidneys, but significant amounts are eliminated in the bile.

Deficiency

A precise description of molybdenum deficiency in humans has not been clearly documented. Evidence so far has been limited to a single patient on long-term total parenteral nutrition, who developed hypermethioninaemia, decreased urinary excretion of sulphate and uric acid, and increased urinary excretion of sulphite and xanthine. In addition, the patient suffered irritability and mental disturbances that progressed into coma. Supplementation with molybdenum improved the clinical condition and normalized uric acid production.

Uses

None established.

Adverse effects

Molybdenum is a relatively non-toxic element. High dietary intakes (10–15 mg daily) have been associated with elevated uric acid concentrations in blood and an increased incidence of gout, and may also result in impaired bioavailability of copper and altered metabolism of nucleotides.

Dose

Not established

Further reading

Rajagopolan K.V. (1988) Molybdenum: an essential trace element in human nutrition. *Ann Rev Nutr* **8**, 410–27.

Chapter 37
Niacin

Description
Niacin is a water-soluble vitamin of the vitamin B complex.

Nomenclature
Niacin is a generic term used to describe the compounds that exhibit the biological properties of nicotinamide. It occurs in food as nicotinamide and nicotinic acid. It is sometimes known as niacinamide.

Units
Requirements and food values for niacin are the sum of the amounts of nicotinic acid and nicotinamide. Niacin is also obtained in the body from the amino acid tryptophan. On average, 60 mg tryptophan is equivalent to 1 mg niacin.

Niacin (mg equivalents) = nicotinic acid (mg) + nicotinamide (mg) + tryptophan (mg)/60

Human requirements
Niacin requirements depend on energy intake; values are therefore given as mg/1000 kcal and also as total values based on estimated average energy requirements for the majority of people in the UK.

Dietary Reference Values for Niacin

Age	RNI (mg[1]/1000 kcal)	RNI (mg[1]/d)
1–6 months	6.6	3
7–9 months	6.6	4
10–12 months	6.6	5
1–3 years	6.6	8
4–6 years	6.6	11
7–10 years	6.6	12
Males		
11–14 years	6.6	15
15–18 years	6.6	18
19–50 years	6.6	17
50+ years	6.6	16

Age	RNI (mg^1/1000 kcal)	RNI (mg^1/d)
Females		
11–14 years	6.6	12
15–18 years	6.6	14
19–50 years	6.6	13
50+ years	6.6	12
Pregnancy	No increment	
Lactation	6.6	+2

1. Niacin equivalents (includes total pre-formed niacin and tryptophan divided by 60).
EAR = 5.5 mg niacin equivalents/1000 kcal (all ages).
LRNI = 4.4 mg niacin equivalents/1000 kcal (all ages).
Reproduced and adapted with the permission of the Controller of Her Majesty's Stationery Office.

Intakes

In the UK the average adult diet provides (niacin equivalents): for men, 42 mg daily; for women, 30.9 mg.

Action

Nutritional

As a vitamin, niacin functions as a component of two coenzymes, nicotinamide adenine dinucleotide (NAD) and nicotinamide adenine dinucleotide diphosphate (NADP). These coenzymes participate in many metabolic processes including glycolysis, tissue respiration, and lipid, amino acid and purine metabolism.

Pharmacological

In doses in excess of nutritional requirements, nicotinic acid (but not nicotinamide) reduces serum cholesterol and triglycerides by inhibiting the synthesis of very low density proteins (VLDL), which are the precursors of low density lipoproteins (LDL). Nicotinic acid also causes direct peripheral vasodilatation.

Dietary sources

Food portion	Niacin content^1 (mg)
Breakfast cereals	
1 bowl All-Bran (45 g)	6.5
1 bowl Bran Flakes (45 g)	7.5
1 bowl Corn Flakes (30 g)	5.0
1 bowl Muesli (95 g)	**8.0**
1 bowl Start (40 g)	**10.0**
2 pieces Shredded Wheat	3.0
2 Weetabix	6.0

Food portion	Niacin content[1] (mg)
Cereal products	
Bread, brown, 2 slices	3.0
white, 2 slices	2.5
wholemeal, 2 slices	4.0
1 chapati	2.5
1 naan	5.0
1 white pitta bread	2.5
Pasta, brown, boiled (150 g)	3.5
white, boiled (150 g)	2.0
Rice, brown, boiled (160 g)	3.0
white, boiled (160 g)	2.0
2 heaped tablespoons wheatgerm	1.5
Milk and dairy products	
½ pint milk, whole, semi-skimmed, or skimmed	2.5
½ pint soya milk	1.5
1 pot yoghurt (150 g)	1.5
Cheese (50 g)	1.5
1 egg, size 2 (60 g)	2.5
Meat and fish	
Beef, roast (85 g)	**10.0**
Lamb, roast (85 g)	**10.0**
Pork, roast (85 g)	**10.0**
1 chicken leg portion	**16.0**
Liver, lambs, cooked (90 g)	**18.0**
Kidney, lambs, cooked (75 g)	**11.5**
Fish, cooked (150 g)	**10–15**
Vegetables	
Peas, boiled (100 g)	2.5
Potatoes, boiled (150 g)	1.5
1 small can baked beans (200 g)	2.6
Chickpeas, cooked (105 g)	2.0
Red kidney beans (105 g)	2.0
Dahl, lentil (150 g)	1.5
Nuts	
30 peanuts	6.5
Yeast	
Brewer's Yeast (10 g)	1.5
Marmite, spread on 1 slice bread	3.5

1. Niacin equivalents (includes both pre-formed niacin and niacin obtained from tryptophan).
Excellent sources (**bold**); good sources (*italics*).
Information derived from *The Composition of Foods*, 5th Edition (1991) is reproduced with the permission of The Royal Society of Chemistry and the Controller of Her Majesty's Stationery Office.

Metabolism

Absorption
Both nicotinamide and nicotinic acid are absorbed in the duodenum by facilitated diffusion (at low concentrations) and by passive diffusion (at high concentrations).

Distribution
Conversion of niacin to its coenzymes occurs in most tissues.

Elimination
Elimination occurs mainly in the urine. Niacin appears in breast milk.

Bioavailability
Niacin is remarkably stable and can withstand reasonable periods of heating, cooking and storage with little loss. Bioavailability of niacin from cereals may be low, but much of the niacin in breakfast cereals comes from fully available synthetic niacin added to fortify such products.

Deficiency
Niacin deficiency (rare in the UK) may lead to pellagra. Early signs of deficiency are vague and non-specific and may include:

- reduced appetite,
- weight loss,
- gastro-intestinal discomfort,
- weakness,
- irritability, and
- inability to concentrate.

Signs of more advanced deficiency include:

- sore mouth,
- glossitis, and stomatitis.

The severe deficiency state of pellagra is characterized by:

- dermatitis (predominantly in the areas of skin exposed to sunlight),
- dementia (associated with confusion, disorientation, seizures and hallucinations), and
- diarrhoea.

Uses
Despite claims made for niacin, it is of unproven value in arthritis, alcohol dependence, schizophrenia and other mental disorders unrelated to niacin deficiency. Nicotinic acid is prescribable on the NHS for hyperlipidaemia, but should not be sold as a supplement for this purpose.

Precautions/contra-indications
Large doses of niacin are best avoided in:

- diabetes mellitus (blood glucose should be monitored);
- gout (may increase uric acid levels);

- peptic ulcer (large doses may activate an ulcer);
- liver disease (large doses cause deterioration).

Supplements containing nicotinic acid should not be used as a cholesterol-lowering agent without medical advice.

Pregnancy and breast-feeding
No problems reported.

Adverse effects
Both nicotinamide and nicotinic acid can be toxic in excessive amounts, but the effects are somewhat different.

Nicotinamide
In normal doses, nicotinamide is not toxic, but chronic administration at doses of 3 g daily for periods greater than 3 months may cause:

- nausea,
- headaches,
- heartburn,
- fatigue,
- sore throat,
- dry hair,
- dry skin, and
- blurred vision.

Nicotinic acid
- Acute flushing (at doses of 100–200 mg but reduced risk with sustained-release preparation);
- pounding headache, dizziness, nausea, vomiting, pruritus;
- occasionally decreased glucose tolerance and increased uric acid levels;
- rarely hepatic impairment (risk may be increased with sustained-release preparations) and
- hypertension.

Interactions

Drugs
Lipid lowering drugs: increased risk of rhabdomyolysis and myopathy (combined therapy should include careful monitoring).

Nutrients
Adequate amounts of all B vitamins are required for optimal functioning; deficiency or excess of one B vitamin may lead to abnormalities in the metabolism of another.

Interference with diagnostic tests
Niacin (high doses only) may interfere with the tests for:

- blood uric acid (may be increased);
- thyroid function tests;
- urinary catecholamines (measured by fluorimetry); and
- urinary glucose (false positive with analyses using cupric sulphate e.g. Clinitest).

Dose

As a dietary supplement, up to 50 mg daily. (Nicotinamide is preferable to nicotinic acid as it does not cause vasodilatation.)

Chapter 38
Pangamic Acid

Description and nomenclature

An alternative name for pangamic acid is vitamin B_{15}, but it is not an officially recognized vitamin.

Constituents

The composition of supplements is undefined but they may contain one or more of the following substances:

- calcium gluconate, glycine,
- NN-dimethylglycine and
- N,N-diisopropylamine dichloroacetate.

   (N,N-diisopropylamine dichloroacetate has pharmacological activity.)

Dietary sources

Apricot kernels, brewer's yeast, liver, wheatgerm, bran and wholegrains.

Uses

Pangamic acid is claimed to enhance athletic performance and to be beneficial in cardiovascular disease, asthma and diabetes mellitus. Scientific studies show no evidence of therapeutic efficacy for pangamic acid.

Adverse effects

Pangamic acid may be mutagenic and thus potentially able to cause cancer. It may cause occasional transient flushing of the skin.

Dose

Pangamic acid is best avoided. Dietary supplements provide 50–100 mg per dose.

Chapter 39
Pantothenic Acid

Description
Pantothenic acid is a water-soluble vitamin of the vitamin B complex.

Human requirements
No Reference Nutrient Intake or Estimated Average Requirement has been set for pantothenic acid in the UK but a safe and adequate intake is: adults, 3–7 mg daily; children, 1–7 mg daily.

Intakes
In the UK the average adult diet provides 5.1 mg daily.

Action
Pantothenic acid functions mainly as a component of coenzyme A and acyl carrier protein. Coenzyme A has a central role as a cofactor for enzymes involved in the metabolism of lipids, carbohydrates and proteins; it is also required for the synthesis of cholesterol, steroid hormones, acetylcholine and porphyrins. As a component of acyl carrier protein, pantothenic acid is involved in various transfer reactions and in the assembly of acetate units into longer chain fatty acids.

Dietary sources

Food portion	Pantothenic acid content (mg)
Breakfast cereals	
1 bowl All-Bran (45 g)	0.7
1 bowl Bran Flakes (45 g)	0.7
1 bowl Corn Flakes (30 g)	0.1
1 bowl Muesli (95 g)	**1.1**
2 pieces Shredded Wheat	0.4
2 Weetabix	0.3
Cereal products	
Bread, brown, 2 slices	0.2
white, 2 slices	0.2
wholemeal, 2 slices	0.4
1 chapati	0.1
Milk and dairy products	
½ pint milk, whole, semi-skimmed or skimmed	0.8
1 pot yoghurt (150 g)	0.6
Cheese (50 g)	0.2
1 egg, size 2 (60 g)	**1.0**

Food portion	Pantothenic acid content (mg)
Meat and fish	
Beef, roast (85 g)	0.5
Lamb, roast (85 g)	0.5
Pork, roast (85 g)	0.8
1 chicken leg portion	**1.5**
Liver, lambs, cooked (90 g)	**7.0**
Kidney, lambs, cooked (75 g)	**4.0**
Fish, cooked (150 g)	0.5
Vegetables	
1 small can baked beans (200 g)	0.4
Chickpeas, cooked (105 g)	0.3
Red kidney beans (105 g)	0.2
Peas, boiled (100 g)	0.1
Potatoes, boiled (150 g)	0.6
Green vegetables, average, boiled (100 g)	0.2
Fruit	
1 banana	0.5
1 orange	0.6
Nuts	
30 peanuts	0.7
Yeast	
Brewer's Yeast (10 g)	**1.0**

Excellent sources (> 1 mg/portion) (**bold**).
Information derived from *The Composition of Foods*, 5th Edition (1991) is reproduced with the permission of The Royal Society of Chemistry and the Controller of Her Majesty's Stationery Office.

Metabolism

Absorption
Absorption occurs in the small intestine.

Distribution
Pantothenic acid is widely distributed in body tissues (particularly in the liver, adrenal glands, heart and kidneys) mainly as coenzyme A.

Elimination
About 70% is excreted unchanged in the urine and 30% in the faeces.

Bioavailability
Bioavailability may be reduced by some drugs (see Interactions) or a high fat intake, and increased by a diet high in protein.

Deficiency
Deficiency has not been clearly identified in humans consuming a mixed diet.

Uses

Rheumatoid arthritis

Pantothenic acid has been claimed to be of value in rheumatoid arthritis. In a clinical trial (General Practitioner Research Group 1980) large doses of calcium pantothenate (500 mg/d) for 8 weeks showed no benefit over placebo treatment on the course of development of rheumatoid arthritis, but were effective in reducing the degree of morning stiffness, the degree of disability and severity of pain.

Pantothenic acid has been used for:

- psychiatric states;
- impaired mental function;
- grey hair;
- increasing gastro-intestinal peristalsis; and
- in the relief of itching in dermatitis,

- alopecia;
- catarrhal respiratory disorders;
- diabetic neuropathy;

but there is no evidence for its efficacy in these conditions.

Adverse effects

No adverse effects except for occasional diarrhoea have been reported in humans.

Interactions

Drugs

Alcohol: excessive alcohol intake may increase requirement for pantothenic acid.

Oral contraceptives: may increase requirement for pantothenic acid.

Nutrients

Adequate amounts of all B vitamins are required for optimal functioning; deficiency or excess of one B vitamin may lead to abnormalities in the metabolism of another.

Dose

Adults and children, up to 100 mg daily.

References

General Practitioner Research Group (1980) Calcium pantothenate in arthritic conditions. *Practitioner* **224**, 208.

Chapter 40
Para-amino benzoic Acid

Description and nomenclature

Para-amino benzoic acid (PABA) is a member of the B complex, but is not an officially recognized vitamin.

Dietary sources

Brewer's yeast, liver, wheatgerm, bran and wholegrains.

Uses

Para-amino benzoic acid is claimed to prevent greying hair and to be useful as an anti-aging supplement. It has been used in digestive disorders, arthritis, insomnia and depression. There is no convincing scientific evidence available.

A derivative of PABA is used topically as a sunscreen agent; this is effective in the prevention of sunburn.

Adverse effects

Toxicity is low, but high doses (> 30 mg) may cause:

- anorexia,
- nausea,
- vomiting,
- liver toxicity,

- fever,
- itching, and
- skin rash.

Interactions

Sulphonamides: kill bacteria by mimicking PABA; supplements containing PABA should be avoided while taking these drugs.

Dose

Best avoided. Dietary supplements provide 100–500 mg per dose.

Chapter 41
Potassium

Description
Potassium is an essential mineral.

Human requirements

Dietary Reference Values (mg/d)

Age	RNI	LRNI
0–3 months	800	400
4–6 months	850	400
7–9 months	700	400
10–12 months	700	450
1–3 years	800	450
4–6 years	1100	600
7–10 years	2000	950
11–14 years	3100	1600
15–50+ years	3500	2000

Note: No EAR has been derived for potassium
Reproduced and adapted with the permission of the Controller of Her Majesty's Stationery Office

Intakes
In the UK the average adult diet provides: for men, 3279 mg daily; for women, 2562 mg.

Action
Potassium is the principal intracellular cation and is fundamental to the regulation of acid-base and water balance. It contributes to transmission of nerve impulses, control of skeletal muscle contractility and maintenance of blood pressure.

Dietary sources

Food portion	Potassium content (mg)
Breakfast cereals	
1 bowl All-Bran (45 g)	450
1 bowl Bran Flakes (45 g)	250
1 bowl Corn Flakes (30 g)	30
1 bowl Muesli (95 g)	500
2 pieces Shredded Wheat	150
2 Weetabix	150

Food portion	Potassium content (mg)
Cereal products	
Bread, brown, 2 slices	100
white, 2 slices	70
wholemeal, 2 slices	160
1 chapati	110
Pasta, brown, boiled (150 g)	200
white, boiled (150 g)	40
Rice, brown, boiled (165 g)	150
white, boiled (165 g)	80
Milk and dairy products	
½ pint milk, whole, semi-skimmed or skimmed	400
1 pot yoghurt (150 g)	370
Cheese (50 g)	50
1 egg, size 2 (60 g)	50
Meat and fish	
Meat, cooked (100 g)	200–300
Liver, lambs, cooked (90 g)	300
Kidney, lambs, cooked (75 g)	250
White fish, cooked (150 g)	400–500
Herring or mackerel (110 g)	460
Pilchards, canned (105 g)	450
Sardines, canned (70 g)	300
Vegetables	
Green vegetables, average, boiled (100 g)	100–200
Potatoes, boiled (150 g)	450
baked (150 g)	950
1 small can baked beans (200 g)	*600*
Lentils, kidney beans or other pulses, cooked (105 g)	300
Soya beans, cooked (100 g)	500
Mixed vegetable curry (300 g)	*1250*
Fruit	
1 apple	100
8 dried apricots	*600*
1 banana	350
½ cantaloupe melon	*750*
10 dates	300
4 figs	*600*
1 orange	300
1 handful raisins	350
Nuts	
20 almonds	150
10 Brazil nuts	200
30 Hazel nuts	250
30 peanuts	200

Food portion	Potassium content (mg)
Beverages	
1 mug hot chocolate	350
1 mug Build-Up	*700*
1 mug Complan (sweet)	*600*
1 mug Horlicks	*600*
1 large glass grapefruit juice	200
1 large glass orange juice	300
1 large glass tomato juice	460

Good sources (*italics*).
Information derived from *The Composition of Foods*, 5th Edition (1991) is reproduced with the permission of The Royal Society of Chemistry and the Controller of Her Majesty's Stationery Office.

Metabolism

Absorption
Absorption occurs principally in the small intestine.

Elimination
Excretion is mainly in the urine (the capacity of the kidneys to conserve potassium is poor); unabsorbed and intestinally-secreted potassium is eliminated in the faeces; some is lost in the saliva and sweat.

Deficiency
Potassium deficiency leads to hypokalaemia, symptoms of which include:

- anorexia, nausea, abdominal distension, paralytic ileus;
- muscle weakness, reduced or absent reflexes, paralysis;
- listlessness, apprehension, drowsiness, irrational behaviour;
- respiratory failure;
- polydipsia, polyuria; and
- cardiac arrhythmias.

Uses

Hypertension
Potassium may lower blood pressure (Cappuccio & MacGregor 1991; Khaw & Thom 1982), but there is evidence of a stronger relationship of the sodium to potassium ratio to blood pressure than that of potassium alone (Grobbee *et al.* 1987). Several other minerals (see calcium, Chapter 9; magnesium, Chapter 34) may affect blood pressure and dietary measures to reduce blood pressure might be more effective if the intake of several minerals is changed simultaneously.

Potassium supplements are seldom required by patients taking small doses of diuretics for hypertension. Potassium-sparing diuretics should be prescribed for the prevention of hypokalaemia in patients taking loop or thiazide diuretics for the treatment of oedema.

Precautions/contra-indications

Excessive doses are best avoided in patients with:

- chronic renal failure (particularly in the elderly);
- gastro-intestinal obstruction or ulceration;
- peptic ulcer;
- Addison's disease;
- heart block;
- severe burns; or
- acute dehydration.

Adverse effects

Nausea, vomiting, diarrhoea, or abdominal cramps may occur, particularly if potassium is taken on an empty stomach. Gastro-intestinal ulceration may result from the use of modified-release preparations. Hyperkalaemia is almost unknown with oral administration provided renal function is normal. Intakes exceeding 17 g daily (unlikely from oral supplements) would be required to cause toxicity.

Interactions

Drugs

ACE inhibitors: increased risk of hyperkalaemia.
Carbenoxolone: reduced serum potassium levels.
Corticosteroids: increased excretion of potassium.
Cyclosporin: increased risk of hyperkalaemia.
Laxatives: chronic use reduces absorption of potassium.
Loop diuretics: increased risk of hypokalaemia.
NSAIDs: increased risk of hyperkalaemia.
Potassium-sparing diuretics: increased risk of hyperkalemia.
Thiazide diuretics: increased risk of hypokalaemia (but potassium supplements seldom necessary with small dose of diuretic).

Dose

As a dietary supplement, no dose established.

References

Cappuccio F.P. & MacGregor D.A. (1991) Does potassium supplementation lower blood pressure? A meta-analysis of published trials. *J Hypertension* **9**, 465–73.
Grobbee D.E., Hofman A., Roelandt J.T., Boomsma F., Schalekamp M.A. & Valkenberg H.A. (1987) Sodium restriction and potassium supplementation in young people with mildly elevated blood pressure. *J Hypertension* **5**, 115–9.
Khaw K.T. & Thom S. (1982) Randomized double-blind crossover trial of potassium on blood pressure in normal subjects. *Lancet* **ii**, 1127–9.

Chapter 42
Riboflavine

Description
Riboflavine is a water-soluble vitamin of the vitamin B complex.

Nomenclature
Riboflavine is the British Approved Name for use on pharmaceutical labels. Riboflavin is used to describe the vitamin in food. It is known also as vitamin B_2.

Human requirements

Dietary Reference Values for Riboflavin (mg/d)

Age	RNI	EAR	LRNI
0–12 months	0.4	0.3	0.2
1–3 years	0.6	0.5	0.3
4–6 years	0.8	0.6	0.4
7–10 years	1.0	0.8	0.5
Males			
11–14 years	1.2	1.0	0.8
15–50+ years	1.3	1.0	0.8
Females			
11–50+ years	1.1	0.9	0.8
Pregnancy	1.4		
Lactation	1.6		

Reproduced and adapted with the permission of the Controller of Her Majesty's Stationery Office.

Intakes
In the UK the average adult diet provides: for men, 2.24 mg daily; for women, 1.89 mg.

Action
Riboflavine functions as a component of two flavin co-enzymes – flavin mononucleotide (FMN) and flavin adenine dinucleotide (FAD). It participates in oxidation–reduction reactions in numerous metabolic pathways and in energy production. Examples include:

- the oxidation of glucose, certain amino acids and fatty acids;
- reactions with several intermediaries of the Krebs cycle;
- conversion of pyridoxine to its active coenzyme; and
- conversion of tryptophan to niacin.

Riboflavine has a role as an antioxidant. It may be involved in maintaining the integrity of erythrocytes.

Dietary sources

Food portion	Riboflavin content (mg)
Breakfast cereals	
1 bowl All-Bran (45 g)	*0.5*
1 bowl Bran Flakes (45 g)	*0.6*
1 bowl Corn Flakes (30 g)	*0.4*
1 bowl Muesli (95 g)	*0.6*
1 bowl Shreddies (50 g)	**1.1**
1 bowl Start (40 g)	**0.8**
2 Weetabix	*0.6*
Milk and dairy products	
$\frac{1}{2}$ *pint milk, whole, semi-skimmed or skimmed*	*0.5*
½pint soya milk	**0.7**
1 pot yoghurt (150 g)	*0.4*
Cheese (50 g)	*0.2*
1 egg, size 2 (60 g)	*0.3*
Meat and fish	
Beef, roast (85 g)	*0.2*
Lamb, roast (85 g)	*0.3*
Pork, roast (85 g)	*0.2*
1 chicken leg portion	*0.2*
Liver, lambs, cooked (90 g)	**3.0**
Kidney, lambs, cooked (75 g)	**1.6**
Fish, cooked (150 g)	*0.2*
Yeast	
Brewer's Yeast (10 g)	*0.4*
Marmite, spread on 1 slice bread	*0.5*

Excellent sources (**bold**); good sources (*italics*).
Information derived from *The Composition of Foods*, 5th Edition (1991) is reproduced with the permission of The Royal Society of Chemistry and the Controller of Her Majesty's Stationery Office.

Metabolism

Absorption

Riboflavine is readily absorbed by a saturable active transport system (principally in the duodenum).

Distribution

Some circulating riboflavine is loosely associated with plasma albumin, but significant amounts complex with other proteins. Conversion of riboflavine to its coenzymes occurs in most tissues (particularly in the liver, heart and kidney).

Elimination

Riboflavine is excreted primarily in the urine (mostly as metabolites); excess amounts are excreted unchanged. Riboflavine crosses the placenta and is excreted in breast milk.

Bioavailability

Riboflavine is remarkably stable during processing that involves heat, such as canning, dehydration, evaporation and pasteurization. Boiling in water results in leaching of the vitamin into the water, which should be used for soups and sauces. Considerable losses occur if food is exposed to light; exposure of milk in glass bottles will result in loss of riboflavine. Animal sources of riboflavine are better absorbed and hence more available than vegetable sources.

Deficiency

Deficiency of riboflavine isolated from other B vitamin deficiencies is rare. Early symptoms include:

* soreness of the mouth and throat,
* burning and itching of the eyes, and
* personality deterioration.

   Advanced deficiency may lead to:

* cheilosis,
* angular stomatitis,
* glossitis (red, beefy tongue),
* corneal vascularization,
* seborrhoeic dermatitis (of the face, trunk and extremities),
* normochromic normocytic anaemia,
* leucopenia, and
* thrombocytopenia.

Uses

Supplements may be required by vegans (strict vegetarians who consume no milk or dairy produce).

   Riboflavine is of unproven value for acne, mouth ulcers, migraine or muscle cramps. At present, there is no convincing scientific data which support its use in human cancer.

Precautions/contra-indications

None

Pregnancy and breast-feeding

No problems reported.

Adverse effects

Riboflavine toxicity is unknown in humans. Large doses may cause yellow discolouration of the urine.

Interactions

Drugs

Alcohol: excessive alcohol intake induces riboflavine deficiency.
Barbiturates: prolonged use may induce riboflavine deficiency.
Oral contraceptives: prolonged use may induce riboflavine deficiency.
Phenothiazines: may increase the requirement for riboflavine.
Probenecid: reduces gastro-intestinal absorption and urinary excretion of riboflavine.
Tricyclic antidepressants: may increase the requirement for riboflavine.

Nutrients

Adequate amounts of all B vitamins are required for optimal functioning; deficiency or excess of one B vitamin may lead to abnormalities in the metabolism of another.
Iron: deficiency of riboflavine may impair iron metabolism and produce anaemia.

Interference with diagnostic tests

Riboflavine (high doses only) may interfere with the tests for:

- urinary catecholamines, measured by fluorimetry (false positive); and
- urobilinogen (false positive).

Dose

As a dietary supplement, 1–3 mg daily.

Chapter 43
Royal Jelly

Description

Royal jelly is a yellow-white liquid secreted by the hypopharyngeal glands of 'nurse' worker bees from the 6th to 12th day of their adult life. It is an essential food for the queen bee.

Constituents

Claimed nutrient composition in a typical daily dose (500 mg) of Royal Jelly

Nutrient	Amount	% RNI[1]
Water (mg)	350	—
Carbohydrate (mg)	60	—
Protein (mg)	60	—
Lipids (mg)	25	—
Thiamine (µg)	2	0.2
Riboflavine (µg)	7	0.6
Niacin (µg)	20	0.1
Vitamin B_6 (µg)	3	0.2
Folic acid (ng)	15	0.08
Biotin (µg)	1	—
Pantothenic acid (µg)	3	—
Calcium (µg)	130	0.02
Magnesium (µg)	150	0.07
Potassium (mg)	2.5	0.07
Iron (µg)	25	0.2
Zinc (µg)	15	0.2

1. Reference Nutrient Intake for men aged 19–50 years.

Action

Royal jelly may have some pharmacological effects, but the only available evidence comes from *in vitro* studies and animal studies. It appears to:

- have anti-tumour effects (Tamura *et al.* 1987);
- improve the efficiency of insulin (Kramer *et al.* 1977);
- have vasodilator activity (Shinoda *et al.* 1978);
- exhibit anti-microbial activity (Fujiwara *et al.* 1990).

Uses

Published papers of the effects of royal jelly in humans are relatively few and many of these are single case histories and not clinical trials.

Royal jelly has been claimed to be beneficial in the following circumstances:

- anorexia, fatigue and headaches (Tamura 1985);
- asthma (Pavlik 1958), (but see Precautions below);
- hypercholesterolaemia (Cho 1977).

Claims for the value of royal jelly in:

- arthritis,
- depression,
- diabetes mellitus,
- dysmenorrhoea,
- myalgic encephalomyelitis (ME), and
- premenstrual syndrome (PMS)

- eczema,
- morning sickness,
- multiple sclerosis,
- muscular dystrophy,

are purely anecdotal and there is no evidence for any of them.

Precautions/contra-indications
Royal jelly should be avoided in asthma (adverse effects reported).

Adverse effects
Allergic reactions (one report of death), and contact dermatitis.

Dose
Not established; dietary supplements provide 250–500 mg daily.

References
Cho Y.T (1977) Studies on royal jelly and abnormal cholesterol and triglycerides. *American Bee Journal* **117**, 36–8.

Fujiwara S., Imaj J., Fujiwara M., Yaeshima T., Kawashima T. & Kobayashi K. (1990) A potent antibacterial protein in royal jelly. Purification and determination of the primary structure of royalisin. *J Biol Chemistry* **265**, 11333–7.

Kramer K.J., Tager H.S, Childs C.N. & Spiers R.D. (1977) Insulin-like hypoglycaemic and immunological activities in honey bee royal jelly. *J Insect Physiology* **23**, 293–6.

Pavlik I. (1958) An experimental treatment of bronchial asthma with royal jelly. *Proceedings of the XVII International Beekeeping Congress 1958*.

Shinoda M., Nakajin S., Oikawa T., Sato K., Kamogawa A. & Akiyama Y. (1978) Biochemical studies on vasodilator factor of royal jelly. *Yakugaku Zasshi* **98**, 139–45.

Tamura T. (1985) Royal jelly from the standpoint of clinical pharmacology. *Honeybee Science* **6**, 117–24.

Tamura T., Fujii A. & Kuboyama N. (1987) Antitumour effects of royal jelly. *Nippon Yakurigaku Zasshi* **89**, 73–80.

Chapter 44
Selenium

Description

Selenium is an essential trace element.

Human requirements

Dietary Reference Values (μg/d)

Age	RNI	LRNI
0–3 months	10	4
4–6 months	13	5
7–9 months	10	5
10–12 months	10	6
1–3 years	15	7
4–6 years	20	10
7–10 years	30	16
11–14 years	45	25
Males		
15–18 years	70	40
19–50+ years	75	40
Females		
15–50+ years	60	40
Pregnancy	60	40
Lactation	75	75

Note: No EAR has been derived for selenium.
Reproduced and adapted with the permission of the Controller of Her Majesty's Stationery Office.

Intakes

In the UK the average adult diet provides 25–129 μg daily.

Action

Selenium functions as an integral part of the enzyme glutathione peroxidase and other selenoproteins. Glutathione peroxidase prevents the generation of oxygen free radicals that cause the destruction of polyunsaturated fatty acids in cell membranes. Selenium spares the requirement for vitamin E and vice versa.

Dietary sources

Food portion	Selenium content (µg)
Cereals[1]	
2 slices bread	**30**
Milk and dairy products	
½ pint milk	3–30
1 egg	3–25
Meat and fish	
Beef, cooked (100 g)	3
Lamb, cooked (100 g)	1
Pork, cooked (100 g)	*15*
Chicken, cooked (100 g)	8
Liver (90 g)	*20*
Fish, cooked (150 g)	**30–50**
Vegetables	
1 small can baked beans (200 g)	4
Lentils, red kidney beans or other pulses, cooked (105 g)	5
Green vegetables, average, boiled (100 g)	1–3
Fruit	
1 banana	2
1 orange	2
Nuts	
20 almonds	1
10 Brazil nuts	**200**
30 peanuts	1

1. Cereals are important sources of selenium, but the content reflects the selenium content of the soils on which they are grown and is therefore highly variable.
Excellent sources (**bold**); good sources (*italics*).
Information derived from *The Composition of Foods*, 5th Edition (1991) is reproduced with the permission of The Royal Society of Chemistry and the Controller of Her Majesty's Stationery Office.

Metabolism

Absorption
Little is known about the intestinal absorption of selenium, but it seems to be easily absorbed.

Distribution
Selenium is stored in red cells, liver, spleen, heart, nails, tooth enamel, testes and sperm. It is incorporated into the enzyme, glutathione peroxidase, the metabolically active form of selenium.

Elimination
Selenium is excreted mainly in the urine.

Deficiency

Deficiency has been associated with muscle pain and tenderness; some cases of cardiomyopathy have occurred in patients on total parenteral nutrition with low selenium status. Keshan disease (which has occurred mainly in China) is a syndrome of endemic cardiomyopathy which is alleviated by selenium supplementation.

Uses

Cancer

Some studies suggest that a deficiency of dietary selenium might increase the risk of cancer in humans (Clark 1985; Shamberger *et al*. 1976). These studies correlated selenium levels in forage crops with corresponding cancer mortality rates by geographical area and found an inverse relationship with cancers at several different sites.

Some investigators have reported that serum selenium concentration in humans is inversely related to cancer risk (Clark & Combs 1986; Salonen 1986). However, serum selenium is not a reliable indicator of long term selenium intake and whether this association is a result of differences in dietary selenium intake or not is unclear. Much of the evidence for a protective effect of selenium in humans is derived from comparisons between subjects with blood levels in the lowest or highest part of the normal range.

It is not yet clear which cancers may be most affected by selenium, although gastro-intestinal and respiratory tumours have been implicated most often. There is not enough evidence to justify the use of selenium supplements in the prevention of cancer at present. Several intervention studies are now in progress.

Cardiovascular disease

Low serum selenium levels have been associated with an increased risk of cardiovascular disease in some studies (Salonen *et al*. 1982, 1985), but not in others (Kok *et al*. 1987; Miettinen *et al*. 1983). The results of these studies are equivocal and the role of selenium in cardiovascular disease remains uncertain.

Miscellaneous

Selenium is of unproven value in hair and nail problems and in arthritis.

Precautions/contra-indications

Yeast-containing selenium products should be avoided by patients taking monoamine oxidase inhibitors.

Pregnancy and breast-feeding

No problems with normal intakes.

Adverse effects

There is a narrow margin of safety for selenium. Adverse effects include:

- hair loss,
- nail changes,
- skin lesions,
- nausea,
- diarrhoea,

- irritability,
- metallic taste,
- garlic-smelling breath,
- fatigue, and
- peripheral neuropathy.

Dose

Not established; 50–100 µg daily is safe. Doses from supplements should not exceed 200 µg daily; intake from all sources (food and supplements) should not exceed 450 µg daily.

References

Clark L.C. (1985) The epidemiology of selenium and cancer. *Fed Proc* **44**, 2584–9.

Clark L.C. & Combs G.F. (1986) Selenium compounds and the prevention of cancer: research needs and public health implications. *J Nutr* **116**, 170–3.

Kok F., de Bruijn A.M., Vermeeren R., Hofman A., van Laar A., de Bruin M., Hermus R.J. & Valkenberg H.A. (1987) Serum selenium, vitamin antioxidants and cardiovascular mortality: a 9 year follow up study in the Netherlands. *Am J Clin Nutr* **45**, 462–8.

Miettenen T.A., Alfthan G., Huttunen J.K., Pikkarainen J., Naukkarinen V., Mattila S. & Kumlin T. (1983) Serum selenium concentration related to myocardial infarction and fatty acid content of serum lipids. *Br Med J* **287**, 517–9.

Salonen J.T., Alfthan G., Huttunen J.K., Pikkarainen J. & Puska P. (1982) Association between cardiovascular death and myocardial infarction and serum selenium in a matched-pair longitudinal study. *Lancet* **2**, 175–9.

Salonen J.T., Salonen R., Pentilla I., Herranen M., Jauhianen M., Kantola R., Lappetelainen R., Maenpaa P.H., Alfthan G. & Puska P. (1985) Serum fatty acids, apolipoproteins, selenium and vitamin antioxidants and the risk of death from coronary artery disease. *Am J Cardiol* **56**, 226–31.

Salonen J.T. (1986) Selenium and cancer. *Ann Clin Res* **18**, 18–21.

Shamberger R.J., Tytko S.A. & Willis C.E. (1976) Antioxidants and cancer. Part VI. Selenium and age-adjusted human cancer mortality. *Arch Environ Health* **31**, 231–5.

Chapter 45
Silicon

Description
Silicon is an ultratrace mineral.

Human requirements
Requirements have not been defined. Silicon may be required by humans, but its nutritional importance has not been established. If humans have a requirement for silicon it is probably in the range of 5–20 mg daily.

Action
Silicon contributes to the structure and resilience of connective tissue and appears to have an important role in the synthesis of bone and cartilage collagen; it may also be involved in bone calcification. The average UK diet supplies about 30 mg daily.

Dietary sources
The richest sources of silicon are wholegrain cereals and root vegetables. Animal foods are poor sources.

Metabolism

Absorption
The mechanisms of absorption are unknown.

Distribution
Silicon is retained mainly in connective tissues, including the aorta, trachea, tendon, skin and bone.

Elimination
Silicon is excreted mainly in the urine.

Deficiency
Silicon deficiency has been described for chickens and rats but more work is needed to clarify the effects of silicon deficiency in humans. Silicon deprivation could have detrimental effects on bone mineralization and brain function.

Uses
Silicon is claimed to be of value in Alzheimer's disease and gastro-intestinal problems, but there is no sound evidence for this.

Adverse effects

Silicon is non-toxic when taken orally.

Dose

Not established.

Further reading

Nielsen F.H. (1993) Ultratrace elements of possible importance for human health: an update. In: *Essential and Toxic Trace Elements in Human Health and Disease: an Update.* (ed. A. Prasad) Wiley-Liss, New York, pp 365–6.

Chapter 46
Spirulina

Description

Spirulina is a blue-green microscopic algae; it grows in fresh-water ponds and lakes, thriving in warm and alkaline environments.

Constituents

Claimed[1] nutrient content of spirulina

Claimed[1] nutrient content of spirulina

Nutrient	per 100 g	per typical dose (10 g)	% RNI[2]
Protein (g)	70	7	—
Fat (g)	7	0.7	—
Carbohydrate (g)	15	1.5	—
Betacarotene (mg)	170	17	—
Thiamine (mg)	5.5	0.5	55
Riboflavine (mg)	4.0	0.4	33
Niacin (mg)	11.8	1.2	8
Pyridoxine (mg)	0.3	0.03	2.5
Vitamin B_{12} (µg)	200	20	1333
Folic acid (µg)	50	5	2.5
Pantothenic acid (mg)	1.1	0.1	—
Biotin (µg)	40	4	—
Vitamin E (mg)	19	0.2	—
Inositol (mg)	35	3.5	—
Calcium (mg)	132	13	2
Magnesium (mg)	192	19	6
Potassium (mg)	1540	154	4
Phosphorus (mg)	894	89	16
Iron (mg)	58	5.8	48
Zinc (mg)	4	0.4	6
Manganese (mg)	2.5	0.2	—
Selenium (µg)	40	4	2

1. Reported on a product label.
2. Reference Nutrient Intake for males aged 19–50 years.

Uses

Controlled studies of spirulina have not been conducted in the UK. Claims emphasize the importance of the chlorophyll content of spirulina. However, chlorophyll is a source of energy for plants and has no known useful function for humans.

Spirulina is claimed to act as a tonic and be beneficial in:

- allergies;
- Alzheimer's disease;
- peptic ulcer;
- increasing stamina in athletes; and
- retarding aging.

There is no evidence for any of these claims. When spirulina was introduced into the USA in 1979 as a slimming aid, the Food and Drug Administration (FDA 1981, 1982) could find no evidence to support these claimed benefits.

Precautions/contra-indications
Spirulina may be contaminated with mercury.

Pregnancy and breast-feeding
Avoid (contaminants – see Precautions).

Adverse effects
Effects not known (contaminants – see Precautions).

Dose
Not established; dietary supplements provide 6–10 g per dose.

References
FDA (1981) Spirulina. *FDA Consumer* **15**, 3.
FDA (1982) Spirulina: a miracle food it's not. *FDA Consumer* **16**, 33–4.

Chapter 47
Superoxide Dismutase (SOD)

Description

Superoxide dismutase is a group of enzymes which is widely distributed in the body; several different forms exist which vary in their metal content. Copper-containing SOD is extracellular and present in high concentrations in the lungs, thyroid and uterus and in small amounts in plasma. SOD containing copper and zinc is present within the cells and found in high concentrations in brain, erythrocytes, kidney, liver, pituitary and thyroid.

Action

SOD enzymes act as scavengers of superoxide radicals, and protect against oxidative damage (by catalyzing conversion of superoxide radicals to peroxide).

Uses

SOD is claimed to be useful for:

- prevention of cardiovascular disease,
- cancer, and
- retardation of aging.

Such claims are probably based on studies which have used SOD by injection in clinical management. SOD is not absorbed from an oral dose and dietary supplements are therefore likely to be ineffective.

Adverse effects

None reported.

Dose

Not recommended as a dietary supplement (ineffective).

Chapter 48
Thiamine

Description
Thiamine is a water-soluble vitamin of the vitamin B complex.

Nomenclature
Thiamine is the British Approved Name for use on pharmaceutical labels. Thiamin is used to describe the vitamin present in food. It is known also as vitamin B_1 and aneurine.

Human requirements

Dietary Reference Values for Thiamin
Note: Thiamin requirements depend on energy intake; values are therefore given as mg/1000 kcal and also as total values based on estimated average energy requirements for the majority of people in the UK.

Age	RNI (mg/1000 kcal)	RNI (mg/d based on EARs for energy)
0–9 months[1]	0.3	0.2
10–12 months[1]	0.3	0.3
1–3 years[2]	0.4	0.5
4–10 years[2]	0.4	0.7
Males		
11–14 years[2]	0.4	0.9
15–18 years[2]	0.4	1.1
19–50 years[2]	0.4	1.0
50+ years[2]	0.4	0.9
Females		
11–14 years[2]	0.4	0.7
15–50+ years[2]	0.4	0.8
Pregnancy[2]	0.4	0.5[3]
Lactation[2]	0.4	0.6

1. LRNI = 0.2 mg/1000 kcal; EAR = 0.23 mg/1000 kcal.
2. LRNI = 0.23 mg/1000 kcal; EAR = 0.3 mg/1000 kcal.
3. Last trimester only.
Reproduced and adapted with the permission of the Controller of Her Majesty's Stationery Office.

Intakes
In the UK the average adult diet provides: for men, 1.95 mg daily; for women, 1.56 mg.

Action

Thiamine functions as a co-enzyme in the oxidative decarboxylation of alpha ketoacids (involved in energy production) and in the transketolase reaction of the pentose phosphate pathway (involved in carbohydrate metabolism). Thiamine is also important in nerve transmission (independently of co-enzyme function).

Dietary sources

Food portion	Thiamin content (mg)
Breakfast cereals	
1 bowl All-Bran (45 g)	*0.4*
1 bowl Bran Flakes (45 g)	**0.5**
1 bowl Corn Flakes (30 g)	*0.3*
1 bowl Muesli (95 g)	*0.4*
1 bowl Porridge (160 g)	0.1
2 pieces Shredded Wheat	0.15
1 bowl Shreddies (50 g)	**0.6**
1 bowl Start (40 g)	**0.6**
2 Weetabix	*0.4*
Cereal products	
Bread, brown, 2 slices	*0.2*
white, 2 slices	*0.15*
wholemeal, 2 slices	*0.2*
1 chapati	*0.15*
1 naan	*0.3*
1 white pitta bread	*0.15*
Pasta, brown, boiled (150 g)	*0.3*
white, boiled (150 g)	0.01
Rice, brown, boiled (160 g)	*0.2*
white, boiled (160 g)	0.01
2 heaped tablespoons wheatgerm	*0.3*
Milk and dairy products	
½ pint milk, whole, semi-skimmed, or skimmed	0.1
½ pint soya milk	*0.15*
Cheese (50 g)	*0.15*
Meat and fish	
3 rashers bacon, back, grilled	*0.3*
Beef, roast (85 g)	0.07
Lamb, roast (85 g)	0.12
Pork, roast (85 g)	**0.55**
1 pork chop, grilled (135 g)	**0.7**
2 slices ham	*0.3*
1 gammon rasher, grilled (120 g)	**1.1**
1 chicken leg portion	0.1
Liver, lambs, cooked (90 g)	*0.2*
Kidney, lambs, cooked (75 g)	*0.4*
Fish, cooked (150 g)	*0.15*

Food portion	Thiamin content (mg)
Vegetables	
Peas, boiled (100 g)	*0.3*
Potatoes, boiled (150 g)	*0.3*
1 small can baked beans (200 g)	*0.2*
Chickpeas, cooked (105 g)	0.1
Red kidney beans (105 g)	*0.2*
Dahl, lentil (150 g)	0.1
Fruit	
1 apple, banana, or pear	0.04
1 orange	*0.2*
Nuts	
10 Brazil nuts	*0.3*
30 Hazel nuts	0.1
30 peanuts	*0.3*
1 tablespoon sunflower seeds	0.1
Yeast	
Brewer's Yeast (10 g)	**1.6**
Marmite, spread on 1 slice bread	0.15

Excellent sources (**bold**); good sources (*italics*).
Information derived from *The Composition of Foods*, 5th Edition (1991) is reproduced with the permission of The Royal Society of Chemistry and the Controller of Her Majesty's Stationery Office.

Metabolism

Absorption

Absorption occurs mainly in the jejunum and ileum by both active transport and also by passive diffusion.

Distribution

Thiamine is transported in the plasma bound to albumin and stored in the heart, liver, muscle, kidneys and brain. Only small amounts are stored and turnover is relatively high so continuous intake is necessary. Thiamine is rapidly converted to its biologically active form (thiamine pyrophosphate – TPP).

Elimination

Thiamine is excreted mainly in the urine. It crosses the placenta and is excreted in breast milk.

Bioavailability

Bioavailability of thiamine may be reduced by alcohol. Thiamine requirements are increased by increasing carbohydrate intake. Thiamine is unstable above pH 7 and the addition of sodium bicarbonate to peas or green beans (to retain the green colour) can lead to large losses of thiamine. It is also destroyed by heat, and by processing foods at alkaline pHs, high temperature and in the presence of oxygen or other oxidants. Freezing does not affect thiamine.

Thiamine antagonists (thiaminases) in coffee, tea, raw fish, betel nuts and some vegetables can lead to thiamine destruction in foods during food processing or in the gut after ingestion.

Deficiency

Thiamine deficiency may lead to beri-beri (rare in the UK). Deficiency is associated with abnormalities of carbohydrate metabolism. Early signs of deficiency (including subclinical deficiency) are anorexia, irritability, and weight loss; later features include headache, weakness, tachycardia and peripheral neuropathy.

Advanced deficiency is characterized by involvement of two major organ systems: the cardiovascular system (wet beri-beri) and the nervous system (dry beri-beri, Wernicke's encephalopathy and Korsakoff's psychosis). Signs of wet beri-beri include enlarged heart with abnormal sinus rhythm (usually tachycardia), and peripheral oedema. Signs of dry beri-beri include mental confusion, anorexia, muscle weakness and wasting, ataxia and opthalmo-plegia.

Uses

Some individuals appear to find thiamine effective as an insect repellant, but controlled trials are required to confirm such an effect. Thiamine is of no proven value in:

- fibrocystic breast disease,
- mouth ulcers,
- diarrhoea,
- fatigue,
- mental disorders,
- neuritis unrelated to thiamine deficiency,
- Alzheimer's disease, or
- multiple sclerosis.

Precautions/contra-indications

None when used as a supplement.

Pregnancy/breast-feeding

No problems reported.

Adverse effects

There appear to be no toxic effects (except possibly gastric upset) with high oral doses. Large parenteral doses are generally well tolerated but there have been rare reports of anaphylactic reactions (coughing, difficulty in breathing and swallowing, flushing, skin rash, and swelling of face, lips and eyelids).

Interactions

Drugs

Alcohol: excessive alcohol intake induces thiamine deficiency.

Nutrients

Adequate amounts of all B vitamins are required for optimal functioning; deficiency or excess of one B vitamin may lead to abnormalities in the metabolism of another.

Interference with diagnostic tests

Thiamine (high doses only) may interfere with tests for:

- serum theophylline,
- uric acid, and
- urobilinogen

Dose

As a dietary supplement, 1–2 mg daily.

Chapter 49
Vitamin A

Description

Vitamin A is a fat-soluble vitamin.

Nomenclature

Vitamin A is a generic term used to describe the compounds that exhibit the biological activity of retinol. The two main components of vitamin A in foods are retinol and the carotenoids.

The term retinoid refers to the chemical entity retinol or other closely related naturally occurring derivatives. These include:

- retinal (retinaldehyde),
- retinoic acid, and
- retinyl esters (e.g. retinyl acetate, retinyl palmitate, retinyl propionate).

Retinoids also include structurally related synthetic analogues which may or may not have retinol-like (vitamin A) activity.

Units

The UK Dietary Reference Values express the requirement for vitamin A in terms of retinol equivalents.

$$\text{Retinol equivalents } (\mu g) = \text{retinol } (\mu g) + \frac{\text{beta-carotene equivalents } (\mu g)}{6}$$

The system of International Units for vitamin A was discontinued in 1954, but continues to be widely used (particularly on dietary supplement labels).

$$1 \text{ retinol equivalent } (\mu g) = 3.3 \text{ units}$$

One unit is equal to:

- 0.3 retinol equivalents (μg)
- 0.3 μg retinol
- 0.3 μg retinol acetate
- 0.5 μg retinol palmitate
- 0.4 μg retinol propionate

Human requirements

Dietary Reference Values for Vitamin A – µg/day retinol equivalent

Age	RNI	EAR	LRNI
0–12 months	350	250	150
1–6 years	400	300	200
7–10 years	500	350	250
11–14 years	600	400	250
Males			
15–50+ years	700	500	300
Females			
15–50+ years	600	450	250
Pregnancy	700		
Lactation	950		

Reproduced and adapted with the permission of the Controller of Her Majesty's Stationery Office.

Intakes

In the UK the average adult diet provides (retinol equivalents): for men, 1834 µg (6052 units) daily; for women, 1606 µg (5300 units).

Action

Vitamin A (in the form of retinal) is essential for normal function of the retina and particularly for visual adaptation to darkness. Other forms (retinol, retinoic acid) are necessary for:

- maintenance of the structural and functional integrity of epithelial tissue and the immune system,
- cellular differentiation and proliferation,
- bone growth,
- testicular and ovarian function, and
- embryonic development.

Vitamin A may act as a cofactor in biochemical reactions.

Dietary sources

Food portion	Retinol (µg)
Cereals	
Breads, grains, cereals	0
Milk and dairy products	
½ *pint whole milk*	*150*
½ pint semi-skimmed milk	55
½ pint skimmed milk	2
½ pint skimmed milk, fortified (various brands)	100–150
2 tablespoons dried skimmed milk, fortified (30 g)	120
Single cream (35 g)	100
Whipping cream (35 g)	*190*
Double cream (35 g)	*200*

Food portion	Retinol (μg)
Hard cheese (e.g. cheddar) (50 g)	*160*
Hard cheese, reduced fat (50 g)	80
Brie cheese (50 g)	*140*
Cream cheese (30 g)	*130*
1 carton yoghurt, low fat (150 g)	10
1 carton yoghurt, whole milk (150 g)	45
Ice cream, dairy (75 g)	90
Ice cream, non-dairy (75 g)	1
1 egg, size 2 (60 g)	*110*
Fats and oils	
Butter, on 1 slice bread (10 g)	80
Margarine, on 1 slice bread (10 g)	80
Low fat spread, on 1 slice bread (10 g)	92
2 Tablespoons ghee, (30 g)	*210*
2 teaspoons Cod Liver Oil (10 ml)	**1800**
Meat and fish	
Bacon, beef, lamb, pork, poultry	Trace
Kidney, lambs, cooked (75 g)	80
Liver, lambs, cooked (90 g)	**20 000**
Liver, calf, cooked (90 g)	**36 000**
Liver, ox, cooked (90 g)	**18 000**
Liver, pig, cooked (90 g)	**21 000**
Liver pate (60 g)	**4400**
4 slices liver sausage (35 g)	**870**
White fish	Trace
2 fillets herring, cooked (110 g)	60
2 fillets kipper, cooked (130 g)	40
2 fillets mackerel, cooked (110 g)	55

Excellent soures (**bold**); good sources (*italics*).
Note: For dietary sources of betacarotene, see carotenoids – Chapter 11.
Information derived from *The Composition of Foods*, 5th Edition (1991) is reproduced with the permission of The Royal Society of Chemistry and the Controller of Her Majesty's Stationery Office.

Metabolism

Absorption

Vitamin A is readily absorbed from the upper gastro-intestinal tract (duodenum and jejunum) by a carrier-mediated process. Absorption requires the presence of gastric juice, bile salts, pancreatic and intestinal lipase, protein and dietary fat.

Distribution

The liver contains at least 90% of body stores (approximately two years' adult requirements). Small amounts are stored in the kidney and lungs. Vitamin A is transported in the blood in association with a carrier, Retinol Binding Protein, (RBP).

Elimination

Vitamin A is eliminated in the bile or urine (as metabolites). It appears in the breast milk.

Bioavailability

Absorption is markedly reduced if the intake of dietary fat is < 5 g daily (extremely rare) and by the presence of peroxidized fat and other oxidizing agents in food. Deficiencies of protein (extremely rare in the UK), vitamin E, and zinc, and excessive amounts of alcohol adversely affect vitamin A transport, storage and utilization.

Deficiency

Vitamin A deficiency is widespread in young children in developing countries and is associated with general malnutrition in these countries. In the UK deficiency is relatively rare (especially in adults).

Symptoms of deficiency include:

- night blindness (due to decreased sensitivity of rod receptors in retina);
- xerophthalmia (can be irreversible), characterized by conjunctival and corneal xerosis, ulceration and liquefaction;
- ultimately severe visual impairment and blindness;
- dryness of the skin and papular eruptions (not a unique indicator of vitamin A deficiency because other nutrient deficiencies cause similar disorders);
- metaplasia and keratinization of the cells of the respiratory tract and other organs;
- increased susceptibility to respiratory and urinary tract infections; and
- occasionally diarrhoea and loss of appetite.

Uses

Children

The Department of Health (1994) advises that all children from the age of 1–5 years should receive supplements of vitamins A and D.

Cancer

A large number of studies have assessed the association between vitamin A and cancer, but not all of them distinguish between retinol (pre-formed vitamin A) and carotenoids. Some case-control studies reporting on the association between pre-formed vitamin A and breast cancer have found modest decreases in risk with higher intake (Katsouyanni *et al.* 1988; London *et al.* 1992; Marubini *et al.* 1988; Zaridze *et al.* 1991) but others (Rohan *et al.* 1988; Toniolo *et al.* 1989; Ingram *et al.* 1991; La Vecchia *et al.* 1987;) have found no association. Prospective data are compatible with a modest protective effect of pre-formed vitamin A (Graham *et al.* 1992; Hunter *et al.* 1993; Rohan *et al.* 1993).

There is some preliminary evidence that pre-formed vitamin A may be modestly protective against colon cancer. Graham *et al.* (1988) found a protective association in a study in New York state. A similar protective effect was observed for women (Heilbrun *et al.* 1989). In a nested case-control study (Comstock *et al.* 1991), subjects in the highest quintile of serum retinol were at reduced risk of colon cancer for up to nine years of follow up. Another study (Potter & McMichael 1986) failed to find any association between colon cancer and vitamin A intake.

Most data suggest that pre-formed vitamin A does not protect against prostate cancer, and an initial study (Graham *et al.* 1983) suggesting an adverse effect has not been confirmed. However, the possibility that higher intakes of vitamin A increase the risk of prostate cancer requires further investigation. The risk of lung cancer may be related to dietary carotene intake rather than retinol (Shekelle *et al.* 1981).

Miscellaneous

There is no evidence of vitamin A being valuable in eye problems or the prevention and treatment of infections unrelated to vitamin A deficiency. Vitamin A supplements have no proven benefits in skin problems (e.g. acne), but synthetic retinoids may be prescribed for this purpose.

Pregnancy/breast-feeding

Excessive doses may be teratogenic (Pinnock & Alderman 1992; Underwood 1989). Doses of 7500 µg (25 000 units) daily during early pregnancy can induce spontaneous abortions and major foetal malformations, including abnormalities of the cranium, face and thymus, congenital heart disease, kidney defects and disorders of the central nervous system.

The Department of Health has recommended that women who are (or may become) pregnant should not take dietary supplements which contain vitamin A (including fish liver oil), except on the advice of a doctor or antenatal clinic and should also avoid liver and products containing it (e.g. liver pate and liver sausage).

Adverse effects

Acute toxicity

May be induced by single doses of 300 mg retinol (1m units) in adults, 60 mg retinol (200 000 units) in children or 30 mg retinol (100 000 units) in infants.

Signs and symptoms are usually transient (usually occurring about six hours after ingestion of acute dose and disappearing after 36 hours) and include:

- severe headache (due to raised intracranial pressure),
- sore mouth,
- bleeding gums,
- dizziness,
- vomiting,
- blurred vision,
- hepatomegaly,
- irritability, and
- (in infants) bulging of the fontanelle.

Chronic toxicity

Signs of chronic toxicity may appear when there is a daily intake > 15 mg retinol (50 000 units) in adults and 6 mg (20 000 units) in infants and young children.

Signs may include:

- dryness of the skin,
- pruritus,
- dermatitis,
- skin desquamation,
- skin erythema,
- skin rash,
- skin scaliness,
- papilloedema,
- disturbed hair growth,
- fissure of the lips,
- bone and joint pain,
- hyperostosis,
- bulging fontanelle (in infants), and
- headache,
- fatigue,
- irritability,
- insomnia,
- anorexia,
- nausea,
- vomiting,
- diarrhoea,
- weight loss,
- hepatomegaly,
- hepatotoxicity,
- raised intracranial pressure,
- hypercalcaemia (due to increase in activity of alkaline phosphatase activity).

Not all signs appear in all patients and relative severity varies widely in different individuals. Most signs and symptoms disappear within a week, but skin and bone changes may remain evident for several months.

Interactions

Drugs

Anticoagulants: large doses of vitamin A (> 750 µg – 2500 units) may induce a hypoprothrombinaemic response.
Cholestyramine and colestipol: may reduce intestinal absorption of vitamin A.
Colchicine: may reduce intestinal absorption of vitamin A.
Liquid paraffin: may reduce intestinal absorption of vitamin A.
Neomycin: may reduce intestinal absorption of vitamin A.
Retinoids (acitrecin, etreninate, isotretinoin, tretinoin): concurrent administration of vitamin A may result in additive toxic effects.
Sucralfate: may reduce intestinal absorption of vitamin A.

Nutrients

Iron: in vitamin A deficiency, plasma iron levels fall.
Vitamin C: under conditions of hypervitaminosis A, tissue levels of vitamin C may be reduced and urinary excretion of vitamin C increased; vitamin C may ameliorate the toxic effects of vitamin A.
Vitamin E: large doses of vitamin A increase the need for vitamin E; vitamin E protects against the oxidative destruction of vitamin A.
Vitamin K: under conditions of hypervitaminosis A, hypothrombinaemia may occur; it can be corrected by administration of vitamin K.

Interference with diagnostic tests

Vitamin A may interfere with tests for:

- blood glucose,
- serum calcium, and
- serum cholesterol and triglyceride.

High doses (> 1500 µg or 5000 units) may decrease:

- erythrocyte and leucocyte counts

and may increase:

- erythrocyte sedimentation rate (ESR), and
- prothrombin time (PT)

Dose

In the absence of malabsorption or gastro-intestinal disease, the following regular daily intakes (from food and supplements) should *not* be exceeded:

- adult women, 7500 µg (25 000 units)
- pregnant women, 2400 µg (8000 units)
- adult men, 9000 µg (29 700 units)
- infants, 900 µg (2970 units)
- children 1–3 years, 1800 µg (5940 units)
- children 4–6 years 3000 µg (9900 units)
- children 6–12 years, 4500 µg (14 850 units)
- adolescents 6000 µg (19 800 units)

Therapeutic doses may exceed these limits but only under medical supervision. For example, in cystic fibrosis, doses of 1200–3300 µg (4000–10 000 units)/d may be given.

References

Comstock G.W., Helzlsouer K.J. & Bush T.L. (1991) Prediagnostic serum levels of carotenoids and vitamin E as related to subsequent cancer in Washington County, Maryland. *Am J Clin Nutr* **53**, 260S–264S.

DoH (1994) *Weaning and the weaning diet. Report of the Working Group on the Weaning Diet of the Committee on Medical Aspects of Food Policy. Report on Health and Social Subjects No 45.* Her Majesty's Stationery Office, London.

Graham S., Haughey B. & Marshall J. (1983) Diet in the epidemiology of carcinoma of the prostate gland. *J Natl Cancer Inst* **70**, 687–92.

Graham S., Marshall B. & Haughey B. (1986) Dietary epidemiology of cancer of the colon in western New York. *Am J Epidemiol* **128**, 490–503.

Graham S., Zielezny M. & Marshall J. (1992) Diet in the epidemiology of breast cancer in the New York state cohort. *Am J Epidemiol* **136**, 1327–37.

Heilbrun L.K., Nomura A., Hankin J.H. & Stemmerman G.N. (1989) Diet and colorectal cancer with special reference to fiber intake. *Int J Cancer* **44**, 1–6.

Hunter D.J., Mason J.E. & Colditz G.A. (1993) A prospective study of the intake of vitamins C, E and A and risk of breast cancer. *New Engl J Med* **329**, 324–40.

Ingram D.M., Nottage E. & Roberts T. (1991) The role of diet in the development of breast cancer: a case-control study of patients with breast cancer, benign epithelial hyperplasia and fibrocystic disease of the breast. *Br J Cancer* **64**, 187–91.

Katsouyanni K., Willett W. & Trichopoulus D. (1988) Risk of breast cancer among Greek women in relation to nutrient intake. *Cancer* **61**, 181–5.

La Vecchia C., Decarli A., Franceschi S., Gentile A., Negri E. & Parazzini F. (1987) Dietary factors and the risk of breast cancer. *Nutr Cancer* **10**, 205–14.

London S.J., Stein E.A. & Henderson I.C. (1992) Carotenoids, retinol and vitamin E and risk of proliferative benign breast disease and breast cancer. *Cancer Causes and Control* **3**, 503–12.

Marubini E., Decarli A. & Costa A. (1988) The relationship of dietary intake and serum levels of retinol and beta-carotene with breast cancer. *Cancer* **61**, 173–80.

Pinnock C.B. & Alderman C.P. (1992) The potential for teratogenicity of vitamin A and its cogeners. *Med J Aust* **157**, 804–9.

Potter J.D. & McMichael A.J. (1986) Diet and cancer of the colon and rectum: a case-control study. *J Natl Cancer Inst* **76**, 557–69.

Rohan T.E., Howe G.R., Friedenreich C.M., Jain M. & Miller A.B. (1993) Dietary fiber, vitamins A, C and E, and risk of breast cancer: a cohort study. *Cancer Causes and Control* **4**, 29–37.

Rohan T.E., McMichael A.J. & Baghurst P.A. (1988) A population-based case-control study of diet and breast cancer in Australia. *Am J Epidemiology* **128**, 478–89.

Shekelle R.B., Lepper M., Liu S., Maliza C., Raynor W.J., Rossof A.H., Oglesby P., Shyrock A.M. & Stamler J. (1981) Dietary vitamin A and the risk of cancer in the Western Electric Study. *Lancet* **2**, 1185–1290.

Toniolo P., Riboli E., Protta F., Charrel M. & Cappa A.P. (1989) Calorie-providing nutrients and risk of breast cancer. *J Natl Cancer Inst* **81**, 278–86.

Underwood B.A. (1989) Teratogenicity of vitamin A. *Int J Vit Nutr Res (supplement)* **30**, 42–55.

Zaridze D., Lifanova Y., Maximovitch D., Day N.E. & Duffy S.W. (1991) Diet, alcohol consumption and reproductive factors in a case-control study of breast cancer in Moscow. *Int J Cancer* **48**, 493–501.

Chapter 50
Vitamin B$_6$

Description
Vitamin B$_6$ is a water-soluble vitamin of the vitamin B complex.

Nomenclature
Vitamin B$_6$ is a generic term used to describe the compounds that exhibit the biological activity of pyridoxine. It occurs in food as pyridoxine, pyridoxal and pyridoxamine. Thus the term 'pyridoxine' is not synonymous with the generic term 'vitamin B$_6$'.

Human requirements

Dietary Reference Values for Vitamin B$_6$
Note: Vitamin B$_6$ requirements depend on protein intake; values are therefore given as µg/g protein and also as total values.

Age	RNI (µg/g protein)	RNI (mg[1]/d)
0–6 months[2]	8	0.2
7–9 months[2]	10	0.3
10–12 months[3]	13	0.4
1–3 years[4]	15	0.7
4–6 years[4]	15	0.9
7–10 years[4]	15	1.0
Males		
11–18 years[4]	15	1.2
19–50+ years[4]	15	1.4
Females		
11–14 years[4]	15	1.0
15–50+ years[4]	15	1.2
Pregnancy	No increment	
Lactation	No increment	

1. Based on protein providing 14.7% of EAR of energy.
2. EAR = 8 µg/g protein; LRNI = 6 µg/g protein.
3. EAR = 10 µg/g protein; LRNI = 8 µg/g protein.
4. EAR = 13 µg/g protein; LRNI = 11 µg/g protein.
Reproduced and adapted with the permission of the Controller of Her Majesty's Stationery Office.

Intakes
In the UK the average adult diet provides: for men, 2.59 mg daily; for women, 3.48 mg.

Action

Vitamin B_6 is converted in erythrocytes to pyridoxal phosphate and to a lesser extent, pyridoxamine phosphate. It acts as a co-factor for various enzymes which are involved in more than 100 reactions that affect protein, lipid and carbohydrate metabolism. Pyridoxal phosphate is also involved in:

- the synthesis of several neurotransmitters;
- the metabolism of several vitamins (e.g. the conversion of tryptophan to niacin); and
- haemoglobin and sphingosine formation.

Dietary sources

Food portion	Vitamin B_6 content (mg)
Breakfast cereals	
1 bowl All-Bran (45 g)	**0.6**
1 bowl Bran Flakes (45 g)	**0.8**
1 bowl Corn Flakes (30 g)	**0.6**
1 bowl Muesli (95 g)	**1.5**
1 bowl Start (40 g)	**1.1**
2 Weetabix	**0.4**
Milk and dairy products	
$\frac{1}{2}$ pint milk, whole, semi-skimmed or skimmed	0.15
$\frac{1}{2}$ pint soya milk	0.15
Meat and fish	
Beef, roast (85 g)	*0.3*
Lamb, roast (85 g)	*0.2*
Pork, roast (85 g)	*0.3*
2 slices ham	*0.3*
1 chicken leg portion	*0.3*
Liver, lambs, cooked (90 g)	**0.4**
Kidney, lambs, cooked (75 g)	*0.2*
Fish, cooked (150 g)	**0.5**
Vegetables	
Potatoes, boiled (150 g)	**0.5**
1 small can baked beans (200 g)	*0.3*
Fruit	
Half an avocado pear	**0.4**
1 banana	*0.3*
Nuts	
30 peanuts	*0.2*
Yeast	
Brewer's Yeast (10 g)	*0.2*

Excellent sources (**bold**); good sources (*italics*).
Information derived from *The Composition of Foods*, 5th Edition (1991) is reproduced with the permission of The Royal Society of Chemistry and the Controller of Her Majesty's Stationery Office.

Metabolism

Absorption
Occurs mainly by a non-saturable process (absorption is greatest in the jejunum).

Distribution
Vitamin B$_6$ is stored in the liver, muscle and brain. Pyridoxal phosphate is transported in the plasma (bound to albumin) and in erythrocytes (in association with haemoglobin).

Elimination
Primarily in the urine (mainly as metabolites), but excess amounts are excreted largely unchanged. It also appears in breast milk.

Bioavailability
Bioavailability of vitamin B$_6$ is affected by food processing and storage. The vitamin is sensitive to light, especially in acid or neutral solutions.

Deficiency
Deficiency of vitamin B$_6$ does not produce a characteristic syndrome, but as with deficiency of the other B vitamins, symptoms such as dermatitis, cheilosis, glossitis and angular stomatitis may occur. Advanced deficiency may produce weakness, irritability, depression, dizziness, peripheral neuropathy and seizures; diarrhoea, anaemia and seizures are particular characteristics of deficiency in infants and children. Chronic deficiency may lead to secondary hyperoxaluria (increased risk of kidney stone formation) and to hypochromic, microcytic anaemia.

Uses

Carpal tunnel syndrome
Idiopathic carpal tunnel syndrome, with swelling of the synovia and compression of the median nerve by the transverse carpal ligament, has been attributed to pyridoxine deficiency (Ellis *et al.* 1977; Fuhr *et al.* 1989). Several studies have confirmed the efficacy of vitamin B$_6$ treatment (Driskell *et al.* 1986; Ellis *et al.* 1979, 1981). No consistent improvement was found in patients with carpal tunnel syndrome and normal vitamin B$_6$ status (Smith *et al.* 1984). These findings led Byers *et al.* (1984) to suggest that clinical improvement in some patients with carpal tunnel syndrome may be due to correction of unrecognized peripheral neuropathy, which could compound symptoms of carpal tunnel syndrome.

Premenstrual syndrome
Pyridoxine has been reported to be of benefit in premenstrual syndrome (Barr 1984; Day 1979; Kerr 1977), but some researchers have found no significant benefit (Hagen *et al* 1985; Malmgron *et al*. 1987, Smallwood *et al*. 1986). Doses of pyridoxine which have shown beneficial effects have been relatively high (500 mg/day) and these high doses should not be recommended because of the risk of toxicity. However, a good response has

been reported with a dose of 50 mg/day (Mattes & Martin 1982). Studies are complicated by the subjective nature of symptoms in premenstrual syndrome, but current evidence indicates that vitamin B_6 may be helpful in alleviating the symptoms of premenstrual syndrome in some women.

Asthma

Low vitamin B_6 status has been reported in adults with asthma (Delport *et al.* 1988; Reynolds & Natta 1985), and in asthmatic children (Hall *et al.* 1982). This may in part be due to use of theophylline which reduces vitamin B status (Ubbink *et al.* 1990). A supplement of 15 mg of pyridoxine per day reduced side effects of theophylline related to nervous system function (Bartel *et al.* 1994).

Vitamin B_6 supplementation (50 mg/day) reduced severity and frequency of asthma attacks (Reynolds & Natta 1985) and pyridoxine (200 mg/day) reduced the need for asthma medication in children (Collipp *et al.* 1975). These findings are promising and warrant further investigation.

Diabetic neuropathy

It has been suggested that peripheral neuropathy in patients with diabetes is associated with pyridoxine deficiency. Diabetics with symptoms of neuropathy and low vitamin B_6 status were given 150 mg of vitamin B_6 daily for 6 weeks (Jones & Gonzalez 1978). Neuropathic symptoms were eliminated in all subjects. The same dose of pyridoxine gradually alleviated pain in patients with painful neuropathy (Bernstein & Lobitz 1988). In diabetic patients whose vitamin B_6 status was normal, pyridoxine supplementation resulted in no improvement in neuropathic symptoms (Levin *et al.* 1981). Further studies are required to investigate the possible benefits of vitamin B_6 in diabetic neuropathy.

Miscellaneous

Pyridoxine has also been reported to be effective in treating pregnancy sickness (General Practitioner Research Group 1963) and hyperactivity in children (Coleman *et al.* 1979). Further confirmation of these possible therapeutic benefits requires properly controlled clinical trials.

Precautions/contra-indications

Hypersensitivity to pyridoxine.

Pregnancy and breast-feeding

No problems reported with normal intakes. Large doses may result in pyridoxine dependency in the infant. There has been one report of amelia of the leg at the knee in an infant whose mother had taken 50 mg pyridoxine daily during pregnancy.

Adverse effects

These include:

- Peripheral neuropathy;
- unsteady gait;
- numbness and tingling in feet and hands;

- loss of limb reflexes;
- impaired or absent tendon reflexes;
- photosensitivity on exposure to sun;
- dizziness;
- nausea;
- breast tenderness; and
- exacerbation of acne.

Adverse effects usually occur with megadoses only. Doses of 2–250 mg daily, even for prolonged periods, appear to be safe, although pyridoxine dependency has been reported with doses of 200 mg daily for over 30 days and impaired memory with doses of 100 mg daily. Symptoms of peripheral neuropathy have occurred occasionally with doses of 50 mg daily. Areslexia and encephalopathy have been reported in infants given 100 mg daily.

Interactions

Drugs

Alcohol: increases turnover of pyridoxine.
Cycloserine: may cause anaemia or peripheral neuritis by acting as a pyridoxine antagonist.
Hydralazine: may cause anaemia or peripheral neuritis by acting as a pyridoxine antagonist.
Isoniazid: may cause anaemia or peripheral neuritis by acting as a pyridoxine antagonist.
Levodopa: effects of levodopa are reversed by pyridoxine (even doses as low as 5 mg daily); vitamin B₆ supplements should be avoided; interaction does not occur with co-beneldopa or co-careldopa.
Oestrogens: (including oral contraceptives) may increase requirement for vitamin B₆.
Penicillamine: may cause anaemia or peripheral neuritis by acting as a pyridoxine antagonist.
Theophylline: may increase requirement for vitamin B₆.

Nutrients

Adequate amounts of all B vitamins are required for optimal functioning; deficiency or excess of one B vitamin may lead to abnormalities in the metabolism of another.
Vitamin C: deficiency of vitamin B₆ may lead to vitamin C deficiency.

Interference with diagnostic tests

Vitamin B₆ may interfere with tests for urobilinogen (may produce a false positive).

Dose

Pre menstrual syndrome, 10–50 mg daily.
As a dietary supplement, 2–5 mg daily (a dose of 250 mg daily, and preferably 50 mg daily, should not be exceeded).

References

Barr W. (1984) Pyridoxine supplements in the premenstrual syndrome. *Practitioner* **228**, 425–7.

Bartel P.R., Ubbink J.B., Delport R., Lotz B.P. & Becker P.J. (1994) Vitamin B_6 supplementation and theophylline-related effects in humans. *Am J Clin Nutr* **60**, 93–9.

Bernstein A.L. & Lobitz C.Z. (1988) A clinical and electrophysiologic study of the treatment of painful diabetic neuropathies with pyridoxine. In: *Clinical and Physiological Applications of Vitamin B_6* (eds J.E. Leklem & R.D. Reynolds), pp 415–23. Alan R Liss, New York.

Byers C.M., DeLisa J.A., Frankel D.L. & Kraft G.H. (1984) Pyridoxine metabolism in carpal tunnel syndrome with and without peripheral neuropathy. *Arch Phys Med Rehabil* **65**, 712–6.

Collipp P.J., Goldzier S., Weiss N., Soleymani Y. & Snyder R. (1975) Pyridoxine treatment in childhood bronchial asthma. *Ann Allergy* **35**, 93–7.

Coleman M., Steinberg G., Tippett J., Bhagavan H.N., Coursin D.B., Gross M., Lewis C. & DeVeau L. (1979) A preliminary study of the effect of pyridoxine administration in a subgroup of hyperkinetic children: a double-blind crossover comparison with methylphenidate. *Biological Psychiatry* **14**, 741–51.

Day J.B. (1979) Clinical trials in the premenstrual syndrome. *Current Medical Research and Opinion* **6**, 40–5.

Delport R., Ubbink J.B., Serfontein W.J., Becker P.J. & Walters L (1988) Vitamin B_6 nutritional status in asthma: the effect of theophylline therapy on plasma pyridoxal-5'-phosphate and pyridoxal levels. *Int J Vit Nutr Res* **58**, 67–72.

Driskell J.A., Wesley R.L. & Hess I.E. (1986) Effectiveness of pyridoxine hydrochloride treatment on carpal tunnel syndrome patients. *Nutr Rep Int* **34**, 1031–40.

Ellis J., Azuma J., Watanebe T., Folkers K., Lowell J.R., Hurst G.A., Ahn C.H., Shuford E.H. Jr & Ulrich R.F. (1977) Survey and new data on treatment with pyridoxine of patients having a clinical syndrome including carpal tunnel and other defects. *Res Commun Chem Pathol Pharmacol* **17**, 165–77.

Ellis J., Folkers K., Watanebe T., Kaji M., Saji S., Caldwell J.W., Temple C.A. & Wood F.S. (1979) Clinical results of a crossover treatment with pyridoxine and placebo of the carpal tunnel syndrome. *Am J Clin Nutr* **32**, 2040–6.

Ellis J., Folkers K., Levy M., Takemura K., Shizukuishi S., Ulrich R. & Harrison P. (1981) Therapy with vitamin B_6 with and without surgery for treatment of patients having the idiopathic carpal tunnel syndrome. *Research Communications in Chemical Pathology and Pharmacology* **33**, 331–44.

Fuhr J.E., Farrow A. & Nelson H.S. Jr (1989) Vitamin B_6 levels in patients with carpal tunnel syndrome. *Arch Surg* **124**, 1329–30.

General Practitioner Research Group (1963) Meclozine and pyridoxine in pregnancy sickness. *Practitioner* **190**, 251–3.

Hagen I., Neshmein B.I. & Tuntlund T. (1985) No effect of vitamin B_6 against premenstrual tension. *Acta Obstet Gynecol Scand* **64**, 667–70.

Hall M.A., Thom H. & Russell G. (1982) Erythrocyte aspartate aminotransferase activity in asthmatic and non-asthmatic children and its enhancement by vitamin B_6. *Ann Allergy* **47**, 464–6.

Jones C.L. & Gonzalez V. (1978) Pyridoxine deficiency: a new factor in diabetic neuropathy. *J Am Podiatr Ass* **68**, 646–53.

Kerr G.D. (1977) The management of premenstrual syndrome. *Current Medical Research and Opinion* **4**, 29–34.

Levin E.R., Hanscomb T.A., Fisher M., Lauvstad W.A., Lui A., Ryan A., Glockner D. & Levin S.R. (1981) The influence of pyridoxine in diabetic neuropathy. *Diabetes Care* **4**, 606–9.

Malmgren R., Collins A. & Nilsson C.G. (1987) Platelet serotonin uptake and effects of vitamin B_6 treatment in premenstrual tension. *Neurophysiology* **18**, 83–8.

Mattes J.A. & Martin D. (1982) Pyridoxine in premenstrual depression. *Hum Nutr Appl Nutr* **36A**, 131–3.

Reynolds R.D. & Natta C.L. (1985) Depressed plasma pyridoxal phosphate concentrations in adult asthmatics. *Am J Clin Nutr* **41**, 684–8.

Smallwood J., Ah-Kye D. & Taylor I. (1986) Vitamin B_6 in the treatment of premenstrual mastalgia. *Br J Clin Pract* **40**, 532–3.

Smith G.P., Rudge P.J. & Peters T.J. (1984) Biochemical studies of pyridoxal and pyridoxal phosphate status and therapeutic trial of pyridoxine in patients with carpal tunnel syndrome. *Ann Neurol* **15**, 104–7.

Ubbink J.B., Vermaak W.J.H., Delport R., Serfontein W.J. & Bartel P. (1990) The relationship between vitamin B_6 metabolism, asthma and theophylline therapy. *Ann NY Acad Sci* **585**, 285–94.

Chapter 51
Vitamin B$_{12}$

Description
Vitamin B$_{12}$ is a water-soluble vitamin of the vitamin B complex.

Nomenclature
Vitamin B$_{12}$ is the generic term used to describe the compounds that exhibit the biological activity of cyanocobalamin. It includes a range of cobalt-containing compounds, known as cobalamins. Cyanocobalamin and hydroxocobalamin are the two principal forms in clinical use.

Human requirements

Dietary Reference Values for Vitamin B$_{12}$ (μg/d)

Age	RNI	EAR	LRNI
0–6 months	0.3	0.25	0.1
7–12 months	0.4	0.35	0.25
1–3 years	0.5	0.4	0.3
4–6 years	0.8	0.7	0.5
7–10 years	1.0	0.8	0.6
11–14 years	1.2	1.0	0.8
15–50+	1.5	1.25	1.0
Pregnancy	1.5	1.25	1.0
Lactation	2.0		

Reproduced and adapted with the permission of the Controller of Her Majesty's Stationery Office.

Intakes
In the UK the average adult diet provides: for men, 7.7 μg daily; for women, 5.9 μg.

Action
Vitamin B$_{12}$ is involved in the recycling of folate coenzymes and the degradation of valine. It is also required for nerve myelination, cell replication, haematopoiesis and nucleoprotein synthesis.

Dietary sources

Food portion	Vitamin B$_{12}$ content (µg)
Breakfast cereals	
1 bowl All-Bran (45 g)	*0.5*
1 bowl Bran Flakes (45 g)	**0.8**
1 bowl Corn Flakes (30 g)	*0.5*
1 bowl Start (40 g)	**1.0**
Milk and dairy products	
$\frac{1}{2}$ pint milk, whole, semi-skimmed or skimmed	**1.0**
Soya milk	
Gold, $\frac{1}{2}$ pint	**1.5**
Plamil, diluted, $\frac{1}{2}$ pint	**3.2**
1 pot yoghurt (150 g)	*0.3*
Cheese (50 g)	**1.0**
1 egg, size 2 (60 g)	*0.4*
Fats and oils	
Butter, margarine, spreads, oils	Trace
Fortified margarine (vegetarian) (10 g)	**0.5**
Meat and fish	
Meat, roast (85 g)	**1.6**
Liver, lambs, cooked (90 g)	**70.0**
Kidney, lambs, cooked (75 g)	**55.0**
White fish, cooked (150 g)	**1.5–4.0**
2 fillets herring, cooked (110 g)	**9.0**
2 fillets kipper, cooked (130 g)	**8.0**
2 fillets mackerel, cooked (110 g)	**15.0**
Pilchards, canned (100 g)	**12.0**
Sardines, canned (70 g)	**10.0**
Tuna, canned (95 g)	**4.0**
Vegetable protein mixes	
Protoveg Burgamix (100 g)	**3.6**
Protoveg Sosmix (100 g)	**1.8**
Yeast extracts	
Marmite, spread on 1 slice bread	*0.4*
Natex, spread on 1 slice bread	*0.4*
Vecon, spread on 1 slice bread	*0.6*

Note: Plant foods (unless fortified commercially) are devoid of vitamin B$_{12}$, except for the adventitious inclusion of microbiologically-formed B$_{12}$ from water or soil.
Excellent sources (**bold**); good sources (*italics*).
Information derived from *The Composition of Foods*, 5th Edition (1991) is reproduced with the permission of The Royal Society of Chemistry and the Controller of Her Majesty's Stationery Office.

Metabolism

Absorption

Absorption occurs almost exclusively in the terminal ileum by an active saturable process, but large amounts (> 30 µg) may also be absorbed by passive diffusion (a maximum of 1.5 µg may be absorbed from oral doses of

5–50 µg). For normal absorption, the vitamin must bind to salivary hapto-corrin and then to 'intrinsic factor' a highly specific glycoprotein secreted by the parietal cells of the stomach.

Distribution
Vitamin B_{12} is stored mainly in the liver. In the blood, it is bound to specific plasma proteins (transcobalamins).

Elimination
Elimination is via the urinary, biliary and faecal routes. Enterohepatic recycling serves to conserve B_{12}. Vitamin B_{12} appears in breast milk.

Deficiency
Deficiency of vitamin B_{12} leads to macrocytic, megaloblastic anaemia. Symptoms include neurological manifestations (due to demyelination of the spinal cord, brain, and optic and peripheral nerves), and less specific symptoms such as weakness, sore tongue, constipation and postural hypotension. Neuropsychiatric manifestations of deficiency may occur in the absence of anaemia (particularly in the elderly).

Pernicious anaemia is a specific form of anaemia caused by lack of intrinsic factor (not lack of vitamin B_{12} in the diet).

Individuals with a reduced ability to absorb B_{12} develop deficiency within 2–3 years. Strict vegetarians (at risk of dietary deficiency, but with normal absorptive efficiency) may not show signs and symptoms for 20–30 years.

Uses

Vegans
Supplementary vitamin B_{12} may be required by vegans. Vitamin B_{12} is found only in animal products and certain foods fortified with the vitamin (see Dietary sources). If vegans do not regularly consume a source of vitamin B_{12}, they will require a supplement. This applies particularly to vegan women during pregnancy as the infant may suffer deficiency. Breast-fed infants whose mothers do not take a source of B_{12} should be supplemented.

Neural tube defects
One study has suggested that deficiency of vitamin B_{12} may be a risk factor for neural tube defects (Kirke *et al*. 1993). This study showed that in affected pregnancies both plasma B_{12} and folate influenced the maternal red cell folate concentration and were independent risk factors for neural defects. More evidence is required before a definite recommendation can be made.

Multiple sclerosis
Vitamin B_{12} has been used to treat multiple sclerosis because it was thought that vitamin B_{12} might have a role in the formation of myelin, the fatty substance which coats nerve cell axons. However, results of early studies in the 1950s and 1960s were inconclusive and interest in B_{12} as a treatment for multiple sclerosis declined. More recently, case reports have appeared (Middleton & Wells 1985; Reynolds & Linnell 1987; Ranoshoff *et al*. 1990) describing an association between vitamin B_{12} and multiple sclerosis or

clinical syndromes resembling multiple sclerosis. Further studies into the metabolism of vitamin B$_{12}$ in multiple sclerosis are warranted.

Miscellaneous

Vitamin B$_{12}$ has been used for a wide variety of conditions, including neurological and psychological disorders (Hillman 1980), fatigue (Ellis & Nasser 1973) and cutaneous sarcoid (Zucker 1975). There is no scientific evidence for a beneficial effect in any of these conditions.

Precautions/contra-indications

Vitamin B$_{12}$ should not be given for treatment of deficiency until the diagnosis is fully established (administration of > 10 μg daily may produce a haematological response in patients with folate deficiency).

Pregnancy and breast-feeding

No problems reported with normal intakes.

Adverse effects

Vitamin B$_{12}$ may occasionally cause diarrhoea and itching skin. Signs of polycythaemia vera may be unmasked. Megadoses may exacerbate acne.

Interactions

Drugs

Alcohol: excessive intake may reduce absorption of vitamin B$_{12}$.
Aminoglycosides: may reduce absorption of vitamin B$_{12}$.
Aminosalicylates: may reduce absorption of vitamin B$_{12}$.
Antibiotics: may interfere with microbiological assay for serum and erythrocyte vitamin B$_{12}$ (false low results).
Chloramphenicol: may reduce absorption of vitamin B$_{12}$.
Cholestyramine: may reduce absorption of vitamin B$_{12}$.
Colchicine: may reduce absorption of vitamin B$_{12}$.
Histamine H$_2$-receptor antagonists: may reduce absorption of vitamin B$_{12}$.
Metformin: may reduce absorption of vitamin B$_{12}$.
Methyldopa: may reduce absorption of vitamin B$_{12}$.
Nitrous oxide: prolonged nitrous oxide anaesthesia inactivates vitamin B$_{12}$.
Oral contraceptives: may reduce blood levels of vitamin B$_{12}$.
Potassium chloride (modified release): prolonged administration may reduce absorption of vitamin B$_{12}$.

Nutrients

Folic acid: large doses given continuously may reduce vitamin B$_{12}$ in blood.
Vitamin C: may destroy vitamin B$_{12}$ (avoid large doses of vitamin C within one hour of oral vitamin B$_{12}$)

Dose

As a dietary supplement, oral, 1–25 μg/d.

References

Ellis F.R. & Nasser F. (1973) A pilot study of vitamin B_{12} in the treatment of tiredness. *Br J Nutr* **30**, 277–83.

Hillman R.S. (1980) Vitamin B_{12}, folic acid and the treatment of megaloblastic anaemias. In: *The Pharmacological Basis of Therapeutics* (eds Goodman & Gillman). MacMillan, New York pp 1331–46.

Kirke P.N., Molloy A.M., Daly L.E., Burke H., Weir D.G. & Scott I.M. (1993) Maternal plasma folate and vitamin B_{12} are independent risk factors for neural tube defects. *Quarterly Journal of Medicine* **86**, 703–8.

Middleton J. & Wells W. (1985) Vitamin B_{12} injections: considerable source of work for the district nurse. *Br Med J* **290**, 1254–5.

Ransohoff R.M., Jacobsen D.W. & Green R. (1990) Vitamin B_{12} deficiency and multiple sclerosis. *Lancet* **1**, 1285–6.

Reynolds E.H. & Linnell J.C. (1987) Vitamin B_{12} deficiency, demyelination and multiple sclerosis. *Lancet* **2**, 920.

Zucker H.S. (1975) Remission of sarcoid. *Ann NY Acad Sci* **75**, 133.

Chapter 52
Vitamin C

Description
Vitamin C is a water-soluble vitamin.

Nomenclature
Vitamin C is a generic term used to describe the compounds that exhibit the biological activity of ascorbic acid. These include L-ascorbic acid (ascorbic acid) and L-dehydroascorbic acid (dehydroascorbic acid).

Human requirements

Dietary Reference Values for Vitamin C (mg/day)

Age	RNI	EAR	LRNI
0–12 months	25	15	6
1–10 years	30	20	8
11–14 years	35	22	9
15–50+	40	25	10
Pregnancy	50		
Lactation	70		

Reproduced and adapted with the permission of the Controller of Her Majesty's Stationery Office.

Intakes
In the UK the average adult diet provides: for men, 77.9 mg daily; for women, 81.8 mg.

Action
The functions of vitamin C are based mainly on its properties as a reducing agent. It is required for:

- the formation of collagen and other organic constituents of the inter-cellular matrix in bone, teeth and capillaries;
- the optimal activity of several enzymes – it activates certain liver-detoxifying enzyme systems (including drug-metabolizing enzymes) and is involved in the synthesis of carnitine and noradrenaline and the metabolism of folic acid, histamine, phenylalanine, tryptophan and tyrosine

It also acts:

- as an anti-oxidant (reacting directly with aqueous free radicals);
- in the protection of cellular function; and
- to enhance the intestinal absorption of non-haeme iron.

Dietary sources

Food Portion	Vitamin C (mg)
Bread and cereals[1]	0
Milk and dairy products	0
Meat and fish[2]	0
Vegetables	
Broccoli, boiled (100 g)	44
Brussels sprouts, boiled (100 g)	60
Cabbage, raw, (100 g)	49
Cabbage, boiled (100 g)	20
Carrots, boiled (100 g)	2
Cauliflower, boiled (100 g)	43
Courgette, stir-fried (100 g)	15
Cucumber, raw (30 g)	2
Kale, boiled (100 g)	71
Lettuce (30 g)	2
Mange-tout peas, boiled (50 g)	14
stir-fried (50 g)	26
Peas boiled, (100 g)	16
Peppers, green, raw (50 g)	120
Peppers, red, raw, (50 g)	140
Potatoes	
chips (250 g)	27
new, boiled (150 g)	15
old, boiled (150 g)	9
sweet, boiled (150 g)	23
Spinach, boiled, (100 g)	8
2 tomatoes, raw (150 g)	25
Watercress (20 g)	12
Fruit	
1 apple	15
1 banana	16
Blackberries, stewed (100 g)	10
Blackcurrants, stewed (100 g)	115
12 cherries	10
Fruit salad	
canned, (130 g)	4
fresh, (130 g)	20
½ **a grapefruit**	54
Grapes (100 g)	3
Guava (100 g)	230
1 kiwi fruit	60
Lychees (100 g)	45
1 mango	50
½ **melon, cantaloupe**	60
1 slice melon, honeydew	18
1 slice watermelon	20
1 orange	90
4 passion fruits	20
1 slice paw-paw	90

Food Portion	Vitamin C (mg)
Fruit (continued)	
1 peach	**30**
1 pear	*9*
1 slice pineapple	*15*
3 plums	6
Raspberries (100 g)	**32**
Strawberries (100 g)	**77**
1 tangerine	**22**
Beverages	
1 large glass apple juice	*28*
1 large glass grapefruit juice	**60**
1 large glass orange juice	**80**
1 large glass tomato juice	*16*
1 large glass Ribena (diluted)	**120**

1. A few breakfast cereals have added vitamin C (average 10 mg/portion).
2. Liver contains approx. 15 mg/100 g.
Excellent sources (**bold**); good sources (*italics*).
Information derived from *The Composition of Foods*, 5th Edition (1991) is reproduced with the permission of The Royal Society of Chemistry and the Controller of Her Majesty's Stationery Office.

Metabolism

Absorption

Vitamin C is absorbed by passive and active transport mechanisms, predominantly in the distal portion of the small intestine (jejunum) and to a lesser extent in the mouth, stomach and proximal intestine. 70–90% of the dietary intake is absorbed, but absorption falls to 50% with a dose of 1.5 g.

Distribution

It is transported in the free form (higher concentrations in leucocytes and platelets than red blood cells and plasma) and is readily taken up by body tissues (highest concentration in glandular tissue, e.g. adrenals and pituitary); body stores are generally about 1.5 g.

Elimination

The urine is the main route of elimination, but very little is excreted unchanged (unless plasma concentration > 1.4 mg/100 ml). Vitamin C crosses the placenta and is excreted in breast milk.

Bioavailability

Storage and cooking lead to loss of vitamin C through oxidation, and boiling results in leaching of the vitamin into the cooking water (cooking water should be consumed in gravies and soups). Microwaving and stir-frying are the best cooking methods for preserving vitamin C.

Deficiency

Vitamin C deficiency may lead to scurvy. Subclinical deficiency has been associated with poor wound healing and ulceration. Early signs of deficiency may be non-specific and include general weakness, lethargy, fatigue, shortness of breath and aching of the limbs. As the disease progresses, petechiae are often prominent and may appear over the arms after application of a sphygmomanometer.

Signs of advanced deficiency include:

* perifollicular haemorrhages (particularly about the hair follicles);
* swollen, bleeding gums;
* pallor and anaemia (the result of prolonged bleeding or associated folic acid deficiency); and
* joints, muscles and subcutaneous tissue may become sites of haemorrhage.

In children, disturbances of growth occur, and bones, teeth and blood vessels develop abnormally; gum signs are only found in the presence of erupted teeth.

Uses

Many health claims have been made for megadose intakes of vitamin C (i.e. 250–10 000 mg per day), including the prevention and treatment of colds, infections, stress, cancer, hypercholesterolaemia and atherosclerosis. Few of these claims have been tested in controlled clinical intervention trials.

Colds

Since Linus Pauling's claims about the beneficial effects of vitamin C on preventing colds and reducing their symptoms, many studies have investigated the effects of vitamin C on the common cold. Hemila (1992) has reviewed the literature. Some investigators but not others have found diminution in cold symptoms in subjects given pharmacological amounts of vitamin C, but the evidence for prevention of colds and infections is largely negative.

Cancer

It has been suggested that vitamin C may be useful in the prevention of cancer (Blocke & Menkes 1989). Possible mechanisms for this protective effect may be that vitamin C:

* acts as an antioxidant,
* blocks formation of nitrosamines and faecal mutagens,
* enhances immune system response, and
* accelerates detoxifying liver enzymes.

Many epidemiological studies have shown an inverse correlation between vitamin C intake and cancer incidence, but the evidence is largely indirect since it is based on the consumption of fruits and vegetables known to contain vitamin C and other nutrients such as betacarotene and folate. The strongest evidence for a protective effect seems to be for stomach cancer (Bjelke 1978; Risch *et al*. 1985; You *et al*. 1988). The evidence for oesophageal cancer is not as strong. Findings are contradictory for cancers of the lung, breast, colon and rectum.

Coronary heart disease

Epidemiological studies have shown associations between low vitamin C intakes and cardiovascular disease risk (Gaby *et al*. 1991). However, two further epidemiological studies of about 87 000 female and 4000 male health professionals found no effect of vitamin C intakes from diets or supplements on cardiovascular risk (Rimm *et al*. 1993; Stampfer *et al*. 1993).

An association between vitamin C and atherosclerosis has been suggested in studies investigating the relationship between vitamin C and cholesterol. When 1 g of vitamin C was given to healthy young people, cholesterol levels tended to fall (Spittle 1972), but in older people no significant pattern of serum cholesterol change was found. Leucocyte levels were found to be lower in patients with coronary heart disease compared to those in patients without CHD (Ramirez & Flowers 1980).

Vitamin C may also have beneficial effects on blood pressure. Several epidemiological studies have been reviewed by Trout (1991) in which vitamin C status or plasma vitamin C was negatively but significantly associated with both diastolic and systolic blood pressure.

Cataracts

Patients with cataracts have been found to have lower levels of vitamin C in the lens than patients with no cataracts (Chandra *et al*. 1986) and as cataracts develop, the vitamin C content of the lens declines (Lohmann 1987). In a retrospective study, a lower incidence of cataract was found in subjects whose ascorbic acid intake was in the highest quintile compared with those in the lowest quintile (Jaques *et al*. 1987).

Wound healing

Reductions in blood ascorbic acid levels have been reported in postoperative patients (Irvin *et al*. 1978; Shulka 1969). Some researchers suggest that this reduction represents increased need, while others suggest that ascorbic acid is redistributed to the tissues. Tissue ascorbic acid concentration at the site of a wound has been found to increase (Crandon *et al*. 1961). Studies have shown accelerated wound healing with vitamin C supplements (Crandon *et al*. 1961; Ringsdorf & Cheraskin 1982).

There is some evidence that vitamin C is of value in the treatment of pressure sores. In a prospective double-blind controlled study, Taylor *et al*. (1974) demonstrated an accelerated healing of pressure sores after one month's treatment with 1 g of vitamin C daily.

Periodontal disease

There is evidence that vitamin C status is related to periodontal disease. Vitamin C depletion in humans has been associated with significantly increased gum bleeding even though no clinical symptoms of scurvy were observed in any subject (Leggott *et al*. 1986). The degree of gingival inflammation was directly related to ascorbic acid status and a reduction in bleeding was observed with vitamin C supplementation (Leggott *et al*. 1986).

Precautions/contra-indications

Vitamin C supplements should be used with caution in:

- diabetes mellitus (interference with glucose determinations);
- glucose-6-phosphate dehydrogenase (G6PD) deficiency (risk of haemolytic anaemia);
- haemochromatosis;
- renal failure (risk of oxalate stones);
- sickle cell anaemia (risk of precipitating a crisis);
- sideroblastic anaemia; and
- thalassaemia.

Prolonged administration of large doses (> 1g daily) of vitamin C in pregnancy may result in increased requirements and scurvy in the neonate.

Adverse effects

Vitamin C is considered one of the safest of all the vitamins. There appear to be no serious health risks with doses up to 10 g daily, but doses of > 1 g daily are associated with osmotic diarrhoea (due to large amounts of unabsorbed ascorbic acid in the intestine), gastric discomfort and mild increase in urination.

Oxalic acid is a major metabolite of vitamin C and there has been concern about an increased risk of renal oxalate stones with high doses. However, oxalate formation is saturable and there is unlikely to be a risk in healthy people, but doses of vitamin C in renal failure should not exceed 100–200 mg daily.

There have been occasional reports that vitamin C destroys vitamin B_{12} in the tissues and of rebound scurvy after administration of vitamin C is stopped, but such reports remain unsubstantiated.

Prolonged use of chewable vitamin C products may cause dental erosion and increased incidence of caries.

Interactions

Drugs

Vitamin C is important for the optimal activity of some of the drug-metabolizing enzymes, including the hepatic cytochrome P 450 mixed function oxidase system. Large doses (> 1 g daily) of ascorbic acid (but not ascorbates) may lower urinary pH, leading to increased renal tubular reabsorption of acidic drugs and increased excretion of alkaline drugs.

Aspirin: prolonged administration may reduce blood levels of ascorbic acid.

Anticoagulants: occasional reports that vitamin C reduces the activity of warfarin.

Anticonvulsants: administration of barbiturates or primidone may increase urinary excretion of ascorbic acid.

Desferrioxamine: iron excretion induced by desferrioxamine is enhanced by administration of vitamin C.

Disulfiram: prolonged administration of large doses (> 1 g daily) of vitamin C may interfere with the alcohol–disulfiram reaction.

Mexiletine: large doses (> 1 g daily) of ascorbic acid may accelerate excretion of mexiletine.

Oral contraceptives (containing oestrogens): may reduce blood levels of ascorbic acid; large doses (> 1 g) of vitamin C may increase plasma oestrogen levels (possibly converting low-dose oral contraceptive to high-dose oral contraceptive); possibility of breakthrough bleeding associated with withdrawal of high-dose vitamin C.

Tetracyclines: prolonged administration may reduce blood levels of ascorbic acid.

Nutrients

Copper: High doses of vitamin C (> 1 g daily) may reduce copper retention.

Iron: vitamin C increases absorption of non-haeme iron, but not haeme iron. For maximal iron absorption from a non-meat meal, a source of vitamin C providing 50–100 mg should be ingested. Vitamin C supplements appear to have no deleterious effect on iron status in patients with iron overload. Iron administration reduces blood levels of ascorbic acid (ascorbic acid is oxidized).

Vitamin A: vitamin C appears to reduce the toxic effects of vitamin A.

Vitamin B_6: deficiency of vitamin C may increase urinary excretion of pyridoxine.

Vitamin B_{12}: excess vitamin C has been claimed to destroy vitamin B_{12}, but this does not appear to occur under physiological conditions.

Vitamin E: vitamin C can spare vitamin E and vice versa.

Heavy metals

Vitamin C may reduce tissue and plasma levels of cadmium, lead, mercury, nickel and vanadium.

Interference with diagnostic tests

Because ascorbic acid is a strong reducing agent it interferes with all diagnostic tests based on oxidation–reduction reactions. Vitamin C administration (megadoses only: > 1 g daily) may interfere with tests for:

- blood glucose (false negative).
- urinary glucose (false positive with analyses using cupric sulphate, e.g. Clinitest; false negative with analyses using glucose oxidase, e.g. Clinistix),
- occult blood in faeces (false negative),
- serum alanine aminotransferase, and
- serum lactate dehydrogenase;

and may decrease:

- serum bilirubin, and
- urinary pH;

and may increase:

- urinary oxalate, and
- urinary uric acid.

Dose
Supplements contain between 25 and 1500 mg per daily dose.

References
Bjelke E. (1978) Dietary factors and the epidemiology of cancer of the stomach and the large bowel. *Klin Prax Suppl* **2**, 10–17.

Blocke G. & Menkes M. (1989) Ascorbic acid in cancer prevention. In: *Nutrition and Cancer Prevention. Investigating the Role of Micronutrients* (eds T.E. Moon & M.S. Micozzi), pp 341–8. Marcel Dekker, New York.

Chandra D.B., Varma R., Ahmad S. & Varma S.D. (1986) Vitamin C in the human aqueous humour and cataracts. *Int J Vit Nutr Res* **56**, 165–8.

Crandon J.H., Lennihan R. Jr, Mikal S. & Reif A.E. (1961) Ascorbic acid economy in surgical patients. *Ann NY Acad Sci* **92**, 246–67.

Gaby S.K. & Singh V.N. (1991) Vitamin C. In: *Vitamin intake and health, a scientific review* (eds. S.K. Gaby, A. Bendich, V.N. Sing & L.J. Machlin), pp 103–61. Marcel Dekker, New York.

Hemila H. (1992) Vitamin C and the common cold. *Br J Nutr* **62**, 3–16.

Irvin T.T., Chattopadhyay D.K. & Smythe A. (1978) Ascorbic acid requirements in postoperative patients. *Surg Gynaecol Obstet* **147**, 49–55.

Jaques P.F., Phillips J., Chylack L.T., McGrandy R.B. & Hartz S.H. (1987) Vitamin C intake and senile cataract. *J Am Coll Nutr* **6**, 435.

Leggott P.J., Robertson P.B., Rothman D.L., Murray P.A. & Jacob R.A. (1986) The effect of controlled ascorbic acid depletion and supplementation on periodontal health. *J Periodontol* **57**, 480–5.

Lohmann W. (1987) Ascorbic acid and cataract. *Ann NY Acad Sci* **498**, 307–11.

Ramirez J. & Flowers N.C. (1980) Leucocyte ascorbic acid and its relationship to coronary artery disease in man. *Am J Clin Nutr* **33**, 2079–87.

Rimm E.B., Stampfer M.J., Ascherio A., Giovanucci E., Colditz G.A. & Willett W.C. (1993) Vitamin E consumption and the risk of coronary heart disease in men. *New Engl J Med* **328**, 1450–6.

Ringsdorf W.M. Jr & Cheraskin E. (1982) Vitamin C and human wound healing. *Oral Surg* **53**, 231–6.

Risch H.A., Jain M., Choi N.W., Fodor J.G., Pfeiffer C.J., Howe G.R., Harrison L.W., Craib K.J.P. & Miller A.B. (1985) Dietary factors and the incidence of cancer of the stomach. *Am J Epidemiol* **122**, 947–9.

Shukla S.P. (1969) Plasma and urinary ascorbic acid levels in the post-operative period. *Experientia* **25**, 704.

Spittle C.R. (1972) Atherosclerosis and vitamin C. *Lancet* **1**, 798.

Stampfer M.J., Hennekens C.H., Manson J.E., Colditz G.A., Rosner B. & Willett W.C. (1993) Vitamin E consumption and the risk of coronary heart disease in women. *New Engl J Med* **328**, 1444–9.

Taylor T.V., Rimmer S., Day B., Butcher J. & Dymock I.W. (1974) Ascorbic acid supplementation in the treatment of pressure sores. *Lancet* **2**, 544–6.

Trout D.L. (1991) Vitamin C and cardiovascular risk factors. *Am J Clin Nutr* **53**, 322S–5S.

You W.C., Blot W.J., Chang Y.S., Ershow A.G., Yang Z.T., An Q., Henderson B., Xu G.W., Fraumeni J.F. & Wang T.G. (1988) Diet and high risk of stomach cancer in Shandong, China. *Cancer Res* **48**, 3518–23.

Chapter 53
Vitamin D

Description
Vitamin D is a fat-soluble vitamin.

Nomenclature
Vitamin D is a generic term used to describe all sterols that exhibit the biological activity of cholecalciferol. These include:

- vitamin D_2 (ergocalciferol),
- vitamin D_3 (cholecalciferol),
- 1 (OH)D_3 (1 Hydroxycholecalciferol; alfacalcidol),
- 25(OH)D_3 (25 Hydroxycholecalciferol; calcifediol),
- 1,25(OH)$_2D_3$ (1,25, Dihydroxycholecalciferol; calcitriol),
- 24,25(OH)$_2D_3$ (24,25, Dihydroxycholecalciferol), and
- dihydrotachysterol.

Units
1 international unit of vitamin D is defined as the activity of 0.025 µg of cholecalciferol.

Thus: 1 µg vitamin D = 40 units vitamin D
and: 1 unit vitamin D = 0.025 µg vitamin D

Human requirements

Dietary Reference Values for Vitamin D (µg/d)

Age	RNI[1]
0–6 months	8.5
6 months – 3 years	7
4–64 years	0[2]
65+ years	10
Pregnancy	10
Lactation	10

1. Supplements may be required to achieve these levels.
2. If skin is exposed to adequate sunlight.
Reproduced and adapted with the permission of the Controller of Her Majesty's Stationery Office.

Intakes
In the UK the average adult diet provides 2.96 µg daily.

Cutaneous synthesis

Exposure of the skin to ultraviolet rays results in the synthesis of chole-calciferol (vitamin D_3); this is the major source of vitamin D. The amount obtained depends on:

- length of exposure,
- area of skin exposed,
- wavelength of UV light,
- pollution,
- skin pigmentation (higher melanin concentration requires longer exposure to achieve same degree of synthesis), and
- age (the elderly may have approximately half the capacity for synthesis of younger people).

Brief, casual exposure of face, arms and hands to sunlight is thought to be equivalent to the ingestion of 5 µg (200 units) of vitamin D (Haddad 1992). The use of sunscreens may affect vitamin D production; application of a sunscreen with a sun protection factor of 8 can completely prevent the cutaneous production of cholecalciferol. However, this should not discourage the use of sunscreens.

Action

Vitamin D is essential for:

- promoting the absorption and utilization of calcium;
- promoting the absorbtion and utilization of potassium;
- normal calcification of the skeleton;
- maintaining neuromuscular function and various cellular processes.

Along with parathyroid hormone and calcitonin, it:

- regulates serum calcium and phosphate levels as needed and
- mobilises calcium from the bone.

Dietary sources

Food portion	Vitamin D content (µg)
Breakfast cereals	
1 bowl All-Bran (45 g)	0.8
1 bowl Bran Flakes (45 g)	1.0
1 bowl Corn Flakes (25 g)	0.5
1 bowl Frosties (45 g)	1.0
1 bowl Rice Krispies (35 g)	0.7
1 bowl Special K (35 g)	0.9
Muesli, porridge, Shredded Wheat, Sugar Puffs, Weetabix	0
Bread	0
Milk and dairy products	
½ pint whole milk	0.1
½ pint semi-skimmed milk	0.03
½ pint skimmed milk	0
½ pint skimmed milk, fortified (various brands)	0.2–0.5

Food portion	Vitamin D content (μg)
Milk and dairy products (continued)	
2 tablespoons dried skimmed milk, fortified (30 g)	1.0
Hard cheese (50 g)	0.1
Feta cheese (50 g)	0.25
1 carton whole milk yoghurt (150 g)	0.06
1 carton low fat yoghurt (150 g)	0.01
1 egg, size 2 (60 g)	1.0
Fats and oils	
Butter, on 1 slice bread (10 g)	0.25
Margarine, on 1 slice bread (10 g)	*2.5*
Low-fat spread, on 1 slice bread (10 g)	*2.5*
2 tablespoons ghee (30 g)	0.6
2 teaspoons Cod liver oil (10 ml)	**21.0**
Meat and fish	
Liver, lambs, cooked (90 g)	0.5
Liver, calf, cooked (90 g)	0.3
Liver, ox, cooked (90 g)	1.0
Liver, pig, cooked (90 g)	1.0
White fish	Trace
Sardines (70 g)	**5.6**
Tinned salmon (100 g)	**12.5**
Tinned pilchards (100 g)	**8.0**
Tinned tuna (100 g)	**5.0**
2 fillets herring, cooked (110 g)	**20.0**
2 fillets kipper, cooked (130 g)	**20.0**
2 fillets mackerel, cooked (110 g)	**21.0**
Beverages	
1 mug Ovaltine[1] (300 ml)	0.7
1 mug Horlicks[1] (300 ml)	0.7
1 mug Build-Up[1] (300 ml)	*3.0*
1 mug Complan[2] (300 ml)	*1.5*

1. Made with milk (whole or skimmed).
2. Made with water.
Excellent sources (> 5 μg/portion) (**bold**); good sources (> 1.5 μg/portion) (*italics*).
Information derived from *The Composition of Foods*, 5th Edition (1991) is reproduced with the permission of The Royal Society of Chemistry and the Controller of Her Majesty's Stationery Office.

Metabolism

Absorption (dietary source)

Vitamin D is absorbed with the aid of bile salts from the small intestine via the lymphatic system and its associated chylomicrons. The efficiency of absorption is estimated to be about 50%.

Distribution

Vitamin D is converted by hydroxylation (predominantly in the liver) to $25(OH)D_3$; this is the major circulating form of vitamin D. From the liver,

$25(OH)D_3$ is transported to the kidney and converted by further hydroxylation to $1,25(OH)_2D_3$, the metabolically active form.

Synthesis is regulated mainly by circulating levels of $1,25(OH)_2D_3$. When levels of $1,25(OH)_2D_3$ are high, synthesis of $1,25(OH)_2D_3$ is low and vice versa. Synthesis is also stimulated by hypocalcaemia, hypophosphataemia and parathyroid hormone (PTH) and inhibited by hypercalcaemia. A second metabolite of vitamin D is produced in the kidney, $24,25(OH)_2D_3$. Both $1,25(OH)_2D_3$ and $24,25(OH)_2D_3$ may be required for the biological activity of vitamin D.

Vitamin D is transported in the plasma bound to a specific vitamin D-binding protein and is stored mainly in the liver, adipose tissue and muscle. Some vitamin D derivatives are excreted in breast milk.

Deficiency

Deficiency of vitamin D results in:

- inadequate intestinal absorption of calcium and phosphate;
- hypocalcaemia, hypophosphataemia and increase in serum alkaline phosphatase activity; and
- hyperparathyroidism.

Demineralization of bone leads to rickets in children and osteomalacia in adults. Infants may develop convulsions and tetany.

Uses

Requirements may be increased and/or supplements necessary in:

- infants who are breast fed without supplemental vitamin D or who have minimal exposure to sunlight,
- pregnancy,
- breast-feeding (particularly with babies born in the autumn),
- the elderly, whose exposure to sunlight may be reduced because of poor mobility,
- individuals with dark skins, and
- strict vegetarians

The Department of Health (1994) advises that all children from the age of 1–5 years should receive supplements of vitamins A and D.

Osteoporosis

Vitamin D may be useful in the prevention of osteoporosis. The association between vitamin D and bone health has been explored in epidemiological studies. These have yielded ambiguous results.

The results of major clinical trials of calcitriol therapy in women with osteoporosis are conflicting. Aloi *et al.* (1988) found that calcitriol treatment reduced bone loss in women with post-menopausal osteoporosis by increasing calcium absorption and reducing bone resorption. Gallagher & Goldgar (1990) showed that treating post-menopausal osteoporosis with calcitriol for two years was associated with an increase in spinal bone density and total body calcium compared with placebo. Continuous treatment of postmenopausal osteoporosis with calcitriol for three years significantly reduced the rate of new vertebral fractures (Tilyard *et al.* 1992).

Annual injection of vitamin D reduced the incidence of hip and other non-vertebral fractures in elderly people (Heikinheimo *et al*. 1992). In another study (Ott & Chesnut 1989) bone mass decreased to a similar extent in patients given calcitriol and those given placebo. Ott & Chesnut (1989) concluded that calcitriol was not superior to simple calcium repletion as a treatment for post-menopausal osteoporosis.

Whether vitamin D has actions on bone other than the promotion of calcium absorption cannot be determined. However, since serum 25-hydroxyvitamin D levels are often low in this age group and vitamin D improves the absorption of calcium in elderly people, the benefit is likely to be an effect of calcium.

Hypertension
Vitamin D, presumably via calcium metabolism, appears to play some role in regulating blood pressure. Vitamin D analogues have been found to reduce blood pressure in intervention trials (Lind *et al*. 1987, 1988, 1989). It remains to be seen whether a beneficial effect on blood pressure can be derived from an increase in dietary or supplemental vitamin D.

Cancer
There is suggestive, but very preliminary, evidence that vitamin D may have an anticarcinogenic action, particularly in colon cancer and possibly in leukaemia. Prospective data from a 19-year dietary survey (Garland *et al*. 1985) showed that risk of mortality from colorectal cancer was inversely correlated with both vitamin D and calcium consumption. In another prospective study (Garland *et al*. 1989), serum concentrations of 20 mg/ml or more were associated with one third of the risk of developing colon cancer that was associated with lower levels of 25-hydroxy vitamin D. While these findings are promising, there is a lack of clinical evidence for an anticarcinogenic effect of vitamin D.

Miscellaneous
There is no evidence for a value of vitamin D in psoriasis, rheumatoid arthritis, or prevention of nearsightedness.

Precautions/contra-indications
Vitamin D should be avoided in:

- hypercalcaemia;
- renal osteodystrophy with hyperphosphataemia (risk of metastatic calcification).

Vegetarians
Supplements containing vitamin D_3 (cholecalciferol) are obtained from animal sources (usually as a by-product of wool fat) and are not suitable for strict vegetarians (vegans). Vitamin D_2 (ergocalciferol) is obtained from plant sources and can be recommended.

Pregnancy and breast-feeding

No problems reported with normal intakes. There is a risk of hypercalcaemic tetany in breast fed infants whose mothers take excessive doses of vitamin D.

Adverse effects

Vitamin D is the most likely of all the vitamins to cause toxicity; the margin of safety is very narrow. There is a wide variation in tolerance to vitamin D, but doses of 250 µg (50 000 units) daily for 6 months may result in toxicity. Infants and children are generally more susceptible than adults; prolonged administration of 45 µg (1800 units) daily may arrest growth in children. Some infants seem to be hyper-reactive to small doses. There is no risk of vitamin D toxicity from prolonged exposure to sunlight.

Excessive intake leads to hypercalcaemia and its associated effects. These include:

- apathy,
- anorexia,
- constipation,
- diarrhoea,
- dry mouth,
- fatigue,
- headache,
- nausea and vomiting, and
- thirst and weakness.

Later symptoms are often associated with calcification of soft tissues and include:

- bone pain,
- cardiac arrhythmias,
- hypertension,
- renal damage (increased urinary frequency, decreased urinary concentrating ability; nocturia, proteinuria),
- psychosis (rare), and
- weight loss.

Interactions

Drugs

Anticonvulsants (phenytoin, barbiturates or primidone): may reduce effect of vitamin D by accelerating its metabolism; patients on long-term anticonvulsant therapy may require vitamin D supplementation to prevent osteomalacia.

Calcitonin: effect of calcitonin may be antagonized by vitamin D.

Cholestyramine, colestipol: may reduce intestinal absorption of vitamin D.

Digoxin: caution because hypercalcaemia caused by vitamin D may potentiate effects of digoxin, resulting in cardiac arrhythmias.

Liquid paraffin: may reduce intestinal absorption of vitamin D. (Avoid long-term administration of liquid paraffin.)

Sucralfate: may reduce intestinal absorption of vitamin D.

Thiazide diuretics: may increase risk of hypercalcaemia.
Vitamin D analogues (alfacalcidol, calcitriol, dihydrotachysterol): increased risk of toxicity with vitamin D supplements.

Nutrients
Calcium: may increase risk of hypercalcaemia.

Interference with diagnostic tests
Vitamin D may interfere with tests for:

- serum alkaline phosphatase (decrease),
- serum and urinary calcium concentration (increase),
- serum cholesterol concentration (increase),
- serum magnesium concentration (increase), and
- serum and urinary phosphate concentration (increase).

Dose
As a dietary supplement, a dose of 10 µg (400 units) daily should not be exceeded.

References

Aloi J.F., Vaswani A., Yeh J.K., Ellis K., Yasumura S. & Cohn S.H. (1988) Calcitriol in the treatment of postmenopausal osteoporosis. *Am J Med* **84**, 401–8.

DoH (1994) *Weaning and the weaning diet. Report of the Working Group on the Weaning Diet of the Committee on Medical Aspects of Food Policy. Report on Health and Social Subjects No 45.* Her Majesty's Stationery Office, London.

Garland C., Barrett-Connor E., Rossoff A.H., Shekelle R.B., Criqui M.H. & Paul O. (1985) Dietary vitamin D and calcium and risk of colorectal cancer: a 19-year prospective study in men. *Lancet* **1**, 307–9.

Garland C.F., Garland F.C., Shaw E.K., Comstock G.W., Helsing K.J. & Gorham E.D. (1989) Serum 25-hydroxyvitamin D and colon cancer: eight-year prospective study. *Lancet* **1**, 1176–8.

Gallagher J.C. & Goldgar D. (1990) Treatment of postmenopausal osteoporosis with high doses of synthetic calcitriol: a randomized controlled trial. *Ann Intern Med* **113**, 649–55.

Haddad J. (1992) Vitamin D – solar rays, the milky way, or both? *New Engl J Med* **326**, 1213–5.

Heikinheimo R.J., Inkovaara J.A. & Harju E.J. (1992) Annual injection of vitamin D and fractures of aged bones. *Calcif Tiss Int* **51**, 105–10.

Lind L., Wengle B. & Ljunghall S. (1987) Blood pressure is lowered by vitamin D (alphacalcidol) during long-term treatment of patients with intermittent hypercalcaemia. *Acta Med Scand* **222**, 423–7.

Lind L., Lithell H., Skarfors E., Wide L. & Ljunghall S. (1988) Reduction of blood pressure by treatment with alphacalcidol: a double-blind, placebo-controlled study in patients with impaired glucose tolerance. *Acta Med Scand* **223**, 211–7.

Lind L., Wengle B. & Ljunghall S. (1989) Reduction of blood pressure during long-term treatment with active vitamin D (alphacalcidol) is dependent on plasma renin activity and calcium status. a double-blind, placebo-controlled study. *Am J Hypertens* **2**, 20–5.

Ott S.M. & Chesnut C.H. III (1989) Calcitriol treatment is not effective in postmenopausal osteoporosis. *Ann Intern Med* **110**, 267–74.

Tilyard M.W., Spears G.F.S., Thomson J. & Dovey S. (1992) Treatment of post-menopausal osteoporosis with calcitriol or calcium. *New Engl J Med* **326**, 357–62.

Chapter 54
Vitamin E

Description
Vitamin E is a fat-soluble vitamin.

Nomenclature
Vitamin E is a generic term used to describe all tocopherol and tocotrienol derivatives that exhibit the biological activity of alpha tocopherol. Those used commercially with their differing biological activities are shown in Table 54.1.

Table 54.1 Biological activity of commercially used vitamin E substances

Name	Biological Activity
d-alpha tocopherol[1]	100%
d-alpha tocopheryl acetate	91%
d-alpha tocopheryl succinate	81%
d, l-alpha tocopherol[2]	67%
d, l-alpha tocopheryl acetate	67%
d, l-alpha tocopheryl succinate	60%

1. Natural vitamin E.
2. Synthetic vitamin E.

Units
The UK Dietary Reference Values express the requirement for vitamin E in terms of milligrams (mg). The system of International Units for vitamin E was discontinued in 1956, but continues to be widely used (particularly on dietary supplement labels).

1 unit = 1 mg of a standard synthetic preparation of alpha tocopheryl acetate and is equivalent to:

- 1 unit dl-alpha tocopheryl acetate
- 1.36 units d-alpha tocopheryl acetate
- 1.10 units dl-alpha tocopherol
- 1.49 units d-alpha tocopherol
- 0.89 units dl-alpha tocopheryl acid succinate
- 1.21 units d-alpha tocopheryl acid succinate.

Vitamin E activity can also be expressed in terms of alpha tocopherol activity and:

1 alpha tocopherol equivalent = 1 mg natural d-alpha tocopherol
= 0.67 units

Human requirements

No Reference Nutrient Intake or Estimated Average Requirement has been set for vitamin E but a safe and adequate intake is:

- for men, > 4 mg daily;
- women, > 3 mg daily; and
- infants, 0.4 mg per g of polyunsaturated fatty acids.

There is an increased requirement for vitamin E with diets high in polyunsaturated fatty acids (PUFA), but many items high in PUFA (e.g. vegetable oils and fish oils) are also high in vitamin E (see Dietary sources). In general, the requirement for vitamin E appears to be:

- 0.4 mg/g of linoleic acid; and
- 3–4 mg/g of eicosapentaenoic and docosahexaenoic acid combined.

Intakes

In the UK the average adult diet provides 8.3 mg daily.

Action

Vitamin E is an antioxidant, protecting polyunsaturated fatty acids in membranes and other critical cellular structures from free radicals and products of oxidation. It works in conjunction with dietary selenium (a cofactor for glutathione peroxidase), and also with vitamin C and other enzymes, including superoxide dismutase and catalase.

Dietary sources

Food portion	Vitamin E content (mg)
Breakfast cereals	
1 bowl All-Bran (45 g)	1.0
1 bowl Muesli (95 g)	**3.0**
2 pieces Shredded Wheat	0.5
1 bowl Start (35 g)	**6.2**
2 Weetabix	0.5
Cereal products	
Brown rice, boiled (160 g)	0.5
Brown pasta	0
Wholemeal bread, 2 slices	*1.5*
2 heaped tablespoons wheatgerm	**3.6**
Milk and dairy products	
½ pint whole milk	0.08
½ pint soya milk	*1.7*
Hard cheese (50 g)	0.25
1 egg, size 2 (60 g)	0.6

Food portion	Vitamin E content (mg)
Fats and oils	
Butter, on 1 slice bread (10 g)	0.2
Margarine, on 1 slice bread (10 g)	0.8
Low-fat spread, on 1 slice bread (10 g)	0.6
2 tablespoons ghee (30 g)	1.0
1 tablespoon olive oil	1.0
1 tablespoon sunflower seed oil	**10**
1 tablespoon wheatgerm oil	**27**
2 teaspoons cod liver oil	*2.0*
Meat and fish	
Liver, lamb, cooked (90 g)	0.3
Liver, calf, cooked (90 g)	0.4
Liver, ox, cooked (90 g)	0.3
Kidney (75 g)	0.3
Sardines (70 g)	0.3
Tinned salmon (100 g)	*1.5*
Tinned pilchards (100 g)	0.7
Tinned tuna (100 g)	0.5
2 fillets herring, cooked (110 g)	0.3
2 fillets kipper, cooked (130 g)	0.4
Vegetables	
Broccoli, boiled (100 g)	1.3
Brussels sprouts, boiled (100 g)	0.9
Sweet potatoes, boiled (150 g)	**6.5**
2 tomatoes	*1.8*
1 small can baked beans (200 g)	0.75
Chick peas, cooked (105 g)	*1.6*
Red kidney beans, cooked (105 g)	0.2
Fruit	
1 apple	0.4
½ an avocado pear	**3.0**
1 banana	0.3
Blackberries, stewed (100 g)	*2.0*
1 orange	0.3
3 plums	0.6
Nuts	
20 almonds	**4.8**
10 Brazil nuts	*2.5*
30 Hazel nuts	**6.2**
30 peanuts	**3.3**
1 tablespoon sunflower seeds	**7.5**
Peanut butter, on 1 slice bread (10 g)	0.5

Excellent sources (> 3.0 mg /portion) (**bold**); good sources (> 1.5 mg/portion) (*italics*).
Information derived from *The Composition of Foods*, 5th Edition (1991) is reproduced with the permission of The Royal Society of Chemistry and the Controller of Her Majesty's Stationery Office.

Metabolism

Absorption

Absorption of vitamin E is relatively inefficient (20–80%); the efficiency of absorption falls as the dose increases. Normal bile and pancreatic secretion are essential for maximal absorption. Absorption is maximal in the median part of the intestine; it is not absorbed in the large intestine to any great extent.

Distribution

Vitamin E is taken up principally via the lymphatic system and is transported in the blood bound to lipoproteins. More than 90% is carried by the LDL fraction. There is some evidence that a greater proportion is transported by the HDL fraction in females than in males. Vitamin E is stored in all fatty tissues, in particular adipose tissue, liver and muscle.

Elimination

The major route of elimination is the faeces; usually less than 1% of orally administered vitamin E is excreted in the urine. Vitamin E appears in breast milk.

Bioavailability

Absorption is affected by dietary fat; medium chain triglycerides enhance absorption whereas polyunsaturated fats are inhibitory.

Vitamin E is not very stable; significant losses from food may occur during storage and cooking. Losses also occur during food processing particularly if there is significant exposure to heat and oxygen. There can be appreciable losses of vitamin E from vegetable oils during cooking.

Water-miscible preparations are superior to fat-soluble preparations in oral treatment of patients with fat malabsorption syndromes. The bioavailability of natural vitamin E is greater than that of synthetic vitamin E (see Table 54.1).

Deficiency

Deficiency of vitamin E is not generally recognized as a clearly definable syndrome. In premature infants, deficiency is associated with:

- haemolytic anaemia,
- thrombocytosis,
- increased platelet aggregation,
- intraventricular haemorrhage, and
- increased risk of retinopathy.

The only children and adults who show clinical signs of vitamin E deficiency are those with severe malabsorption (i.e. in abetalipoproteinaemia, chronic cholestasis, biliary atresia and cystic fibrosis), or those with familial isolated vitamin E deficiency (rare inborn error of vitamin E metabolism). Clinical signs of deficiency include:

- axonal dystrophy,
- reduced red blood cell half-life, and

- neuromuscular disturbances.

Uses

A large number of claims for vitamin E have been made, but they are generally difficult to evaluate since they are often anecdotal or deduced from poorly designed trials.

Cancer

Vitamin E has been suggested to be protective against cancer, an association which has been reviewed by Block (1992) and Knekt (1993). Several epidemiological studies have found lower serum levels of vitamin E in patients who have cancer than those people without cancer. Wald *et al.* (1984) found that the lowest serum levels of vitamin E were associated with a five-fold increase in breast cancer risk compared with the highest levels. Menkes *et al.* (1986) found that the lowest quintile of serum vitamin E level was associated with 2.5 times the relative risk of developing lung cancer compared with the highest quintile. This inverse relationship between serum levels of vitamin E and cancer risk has also been confirmed by Kok *et al.* (1987) and Knekt *et al.* (1988; 1991).

The prospective Iowa Womens' Health Study (Bostick *et al.* 1993) showed that a reduced risk of colon cancer was associated with high intakes of supplemental vitamin E in women under 65 years of age.

However, some studies have not found significant differences in vitamin E status between individuals who later developed cancer and those who did not (Stahelin *et al.* 1984; Wald *et al.* 1987; Willett *et al.* 1984). The Nurses' Health Study (Hunter *et al.* 1993) showed that large intakes of vitamin E did not protect women against breast cancer.

Cardiovascular disease

Platelet aggregation

Vitamin E may decrease platelet aggregation, particularly in diabetic patients. A double-blind crossover placebo study of nine patients with insulin dependent diabetes mellitus treated with 1 g of vitamin E for 35 days showed significant reduction in platelet aggregation (Collette *et al.* 1988). Supplements of 200 units a day reduced *in vitro* platelet activity in women on oral contraceptives (Renaud *et al.* 1987) and 400 units a day inhibited *in vitro* platelet adhesion to collagen in healthy adults (Steiner 1987). In men with low antioxidant status, vitamin E reduced the capacity of the platelets to aggregate (Salonen *et al.* 1991). However, healthy volunteers supplemented with 800 units of vitamin E daily for five weeks showed no significant differences from controls in bleeding times (Stampfer *et al.* 1988).

Intermittent claudication

There is some evidence for a beneficial effect of vitamin E in intermittent claudication (Haeger 1974; Williams *et al.* 1971). Supplements of 300 units of vitamin E daily improved walking distance in treated versus placebo patients (Haeger 1974). Similar results were found in follow-up studies of the use of vitamin E in long-term treatment for intermittent claudication (Haeger 1978, 1982).

Angina

Vitamin E has been claimed to have a beneficial effect in angina pectoris (Shute *et al.* 1948). Randomized, double-blind trials have never supported this assertion (Anderson & Reid 1974; Gillilan *et al.* 1977; Rinzler *et al.* 1950). There is no evidence that vitamin E has any effect in angina pectoris.

Hypercholesterolaemia

Evidence for a beneficial effect of vitamin E in hypercholesterolaemia is scanty. In a study of 10 subjects Hermann *et al.* (1979) found that supplementation with 600 mg vitamin E daily increased HDL cholesterol. However, other studies have never confirmed this effect (Howard *et al.* 1982; Schwartz & Rutherford 1981; Stampfer *et al.* 1983).

Athletic performance

Vitamin E supplementation has been claimed to enhance athletic performance. However, in competition swimmers, Lawrence *et al.* (1975) and Sharman *et al.* (1976) found no significant difference in performance with vitamin E supplementation. Human studies indicate that vitamin E supplementation reduces the oxidative stress induced by exercise. Meydani *et al.* (1993) showed that 48 days of vitamin E supplementation increased muscle alpha-tocopherol and reduced oxidative injury.

Fibrocystic breast disease

Vitamin E may have a beneficial effect in fibrocystic breast disease. Some studies have found clinical improvement in patients treated with 600 mg of vitamin E daily (London *et al.* 1978, 1981; Sundaram *et al.* 1981). Other studies did not find evidence of this beneficial effect (Ernster *et al.* 1985; London *et al.* 1985).

Parkinson's disease

It has been suggested that oxidative damage may be involved in the development of Parkinson's disease and that vitamin E in its antioxidant role may be effective in the early treatment of the disease. A preliminary human trial (Fahn 1989) was encouraging and in another study patients with Parkinson's disease who were taking supplements of vitamin E had significantly less severe disease than matched controls (Factor & Weiner 1989).

Blood disorders

Vitamin E may contribute to the stability of the red blood cell by preventing membrane lipid peroxidation. In doses of 400–800 units daily vitamin E may protect genetically defective blood cells against oxidative damage in patients with glucose-6-phosphate-dehydrogenase deficiency (Corash *et al.* 1980; Spielberg *et al.* 1979) and sickle cell anaemia (Jain 1989; Natta *et al.* 1980).

Cataract

Epidemiological evidence suggests an association between cataract incidence and antioxidant status. Robinson *et al.* (1991) showed that patients with cataracts used significantly less supplementary vitamin E and C than cataract-free patients. Subjects with a low to moderate intake of vitamin E from foods had a higher risk of cataract relative to subjects with higher intakes (Jacques & Chylack 1991). Low serum levels of vitamin E and betacarotene were related to increased risk of cataract in a Finnish study (Knekt *et al.* 1992).

Miscellaneous

Vitamin E has not been proven effective for hair loss, retardation of aging, menopausal syndrome, infertility, impotence or liver spots on the hands.

Precautions/contra-indications

Vitamin E supplements should be avoided:

- by patients taking oral anti-coagulants (increased bleeding tendency);
- in iron deficiency anaemia (vitamin E may impair haematological response to iron); and
- in hyperthyroidism.

Pregnancy and breast-feeding

No problems reported at normal intakes.

Adverse effects

Vitamin E is relatively non-toxic (fractional absorption declines rapidly with increasing intake, thereby preventing the accumulation of toxic concentrations of vitamin E in the tissues). Most adults can tolerate 100–800 mg daily and even doses of 3200 mg daily do not appear to lead to consistent adverse effects.

Large doses (> 1000 mg daily for prolonged periods) have occasionally been associated with the following side-effects:

- increased bleeding tendency in vitamin K deficient patients;
- altered endocrine function (thyroid, adrenal and pituitary); and
- rarely, blurred vision, diarrhoea, dizziness, fatigue and weakness, gynaecomastia, headache and nausea.

Interactions

Drugs

Anti-coagulants: large doses of vitamin E may increase the anti-coagulant effect.

Anticonvulsants (phenobarbitone, phenytoin, carbamazepine): may reduce plasma levels of vitamin E.

Cholestyramine or colestipol: may reduce intestinal absorption of vitamin E.

Digoxin: requirement for digoxin may be reduced with vitamin E (monitoring recommended).

Insulin: requirement for insulin may be reduced by vitamin E (monitoring recommended).

Liquid paraffin: may reduce intestinal absorption of vitamin E (avoid long-term use of liquid paraffin).

Oral contraceptives: may reduce plasma vitamin E levels.

Sucralfate: may reduce intestinal absorption of vitamin E.

Nutrients

Copper: large doses of copper may increase requirement for vitamin E.
Iron: large doses of iron may increase requirements for vitamin E; vitamin E may impair the haematological response in iron deficiency anaemia.
Polyunsaturated fatty acids: the dietary requirement for vitamin E increases when the intake of PUFA increases.
Vitamin A: vitamin E spares vitamin A and protects against some signs of vitamin A toxicity; very high levels of vitamin A may increase requirement of vitamin E; excessive doses of vitamin E may deplete vitamin A.
Vitamin C: vitamin C can spare vitamin E; vitamin E can spare vitamin C.
Vitamin K: large doses of vitamin E (1200 mg daily) increase the vitamin K requirement.
Zinc: zinc deficiency may result in reduced plasma vitamin E levels.

Interference with diagnostic tests

Large doses of vitamin E may increase:

- serum cholesterol concentration,
- serum triglyceride concentration.

Dose

Not established; dietary supplements provide 10–1000 units per daily dose.

References

Anderson T.W. & Reid D.B.W. (1974) A double-blind trial of vitamin E in angina pectoris. *Am J Clin Nutr* **27**, 1174–8.

Block G (1992) The data support a role for antioxidants in reducing cancer risks. Nutrition Reviews **50**, 207–13.

Bostick R.M., Potter J.D., McKenzie D.R., Sellers T.A., Kushi L.H., Steinmetz K.A. & Folsom A.R. (1993) Reduced risk of colon cancer with high intake of vitamin E: The Iowa Women's health study. *Cancer Research* **53**, 4230–7.

Colette C, Pares-Herbute N, Monnier L.H. & Cartry E. (1988) Platelet function in type I diabetes: effects of supplementation with large doses of vitamin E. *Am J Clin Nutr* **47**, 256–71.

Corash L, Spielberg S., Bartsocas C., Boxer L., Steinherz R., Sheetz M., Egan M., Schlessman J. & Schulman J.D. (1980) Reduced chronic hemolysis during high-dose vitamin E administration in Mediterranean-type-glucose-6-phosphate dehydrogenase deficiency. *New Engl J Med* **303**, 416–20.

Ernster V.L., Goodson W.H., Hunt T.K., Petrakis N.L., Sickles E.A. & Miike R. (1985) Vitamin-E and benign breast disease: a double-blind, randomized clinical trial. *Surgery* **97**, 490–4.

Factor S.A. & Weiner W.J. (1989) Retrospective evaluation of vitamin E therapy in Parkinson's disease. *Ann NY Acad Sci* **570**, 441–2.

Fahn S. (1989) The endogenous toxin hypothesis of the etiology of Parkinson's disease and a pilot trial of high-dosage antioxidants in an attempt to slow the progression of the illness. *Ann NY Acad Sci* **570**, 186–96.

Gillilan R.E., Mondell B. & Warbasse J.R. (1977) Quantitative evaluation of vitamin E in the treatment of angina pectoris. *Am Heart J* **93**, 444–9.

Haeger K. (1974) Long-time treatment of intermittent claudication with vitamin E. *Am J Clin Nutr* **27**, 1179–81.

Haeger K. (1978) Long-term observation of patients with atherosclerotic dysbasia on alpha-tocopherol treatment. In: *Tocopherol, Oxygen and Biomembranes* (eds

C. de Duve & O. Hayaishi), pp 319–32. Elsevier/North Holland Biomedical Press.

Haeger K. (1982) Long-term study of alpha-tocopherol in intermittent claudication. *Ann NY Acad Sci* **393**, 369–75.

Hermann W.J., Ward K. & Faucett J. (1979) The effect of tocopherol on high-density lipoprotein cholesterol. *Am J Clin Pathol* **72**, 848–52.

Howard L., Ovesen L., Satya-Murti S. & Chu R. (1982) Reversible neurological symptoms caused by vitamin E deficiency in a patient with short bowel syndrome. *Am J Clin Nutr* **36**, 1243–9.

Hunter D.J., Manson J.E., Colditz G.A., Stampfer M.J., Redner B. Hennekens C.H., Speizer F.E. & Willett W.C. (1993) A prospective study of the intake of vitamin C, E and A and the risk of breast cancer. *New Engl J Med* **329**, 234–40.

Jacques P.F. & Chylack L.T. (1991) Epidemiologic evidence of a role for the anti-oxidant vitamins and carotenoids in cataract prevention. *Am J Clin Nutr* **53**, 352S–355S.

Jain S.K. (1989) Vitamin E and membrane abnormalities in red cells of sickle cell disease and newborn infants. *Ann NY Acad Sci* **570**, 461–3.

Knekt P., Aromaa A., Maatela J., Aaran R-K., Nikkari T., Hakama M., Hakulinen T., Peto R., Saxen E. & Teppo L. (1988) Serum vitamin E and risk of cancer among Finnish men during a 10-year follow-up. *Am J Epidemiol* **127**, 28–41.

Knekt P., Aromaa A., Maatela J., Aaran R-K, Nikkari T., Hakama M., Hakulinen T., Peto R. & Teppo L. (1991) Vitamin E and cancer prevention. *Am J Clin Nutr* **53**, 283S–286S.

Knekt P., Heliovaara M., Rissanen A., Aromaa A. & Aaran R-K. (1992) Serum antioxidant vitamins and risk of cataract. *Br Med J* **305**,1392–4.

Knekt P. (1993) Epidemiology of vitamin E: Evidence for anticancer effects in humans. In: *Vitamin E in Health and Disease* (eds L. Packer & J. Fuchs), pp 513–27. Marcel Dekker Inc. New York.

Kok F.J., van Duijn C.M., Hofman A., Vermeeren R., de Bruijn A.M. & Valkenberg H.A. (1987) Micronutrients and the risk of lung cancer. *New Engl J Med* **316**, 416.

Lawrence J.D., Bower R.C., Riehl W.P. & Smith J.L. (1975) Effects of alpha-tocopherol acetate on the swimming endurance of trained swimmers. *Am J Clin Nutr* **28**, 205–8.

London R.S., Solomon D.M., London E.D., Strummer D., Bankoski J. & Nair P.P. (1978) Mammary dysplasia: Clinical response and urinary excretion of 11-deoxy-17-ketosteroids and pregnanediol following alpha-tocopherol therapy. *Breast* **4**, 19–22.

London R.S., Sundaram G.S., Murphy L., Manimekalai S., Reynolds M & Goldstein P.J. (1985) The effect of vitamin E on mammary dysplasia: a double-blind study. *Obstet Gynecol* **65**, 104–6.

London R.S., Sundaram G.S., Schultz M., Nair P.P. & Goldstein P.J. (1981) Endocrine parameters and alpha tocopherol therapy of patients with mammary dysplasia. *Cancer Res* **41**, 3811–3.

Menkes M.S., Comstock G.W., Vuillemier J.P., Helsing K.J., Rider A.A. & Brookmeyer R. (1986) Serum beta-carotene, vitamins A and E, selenium and risk of lung cancer. *N Engl J Med* **315**, 1250–4.

Meydani M., Evans W.J., Hendelman G., Biddle L., Fielding R.A., Meydani S.N., Burrill J., Fiatarone M.A., Blumberg J.B. & Cannon J.G. (1993) Protective effect of vitamin E on exercise-induced oxidative damage in young and older adults. *Am J Physiol* **264**, R992–S998.

Natta C.L., Machlin L.J, & Brin M (1980) A decrease in irreversibly sickled erythrocytes in sickle cell anaemia patients given vitamin E. *Am J Clin Nutr* **33**, 968–71.

Renaud S., Civatti M., Perrot L., Berthezene F., Dargent D. & Condamin P. (1987)

Influence of vitamin E administration on platelet functions in hormonal contraceptive users. *Contraception* **36**, 347–58.

Rinzler S.H., Bakst H., Benjamin Z.H., Bobb A.L. & Travell J. (1950) Failure of alpha tocopherol to influence pain in patients with heart disease. *Circulation* **1**, 288–93.

Robinson J. McD., Donner A.P. & Trevithick J.R. (1991) A possible role for vitamins C and E in cataract prevention. *Am J Clin Nutr* **53**, 346S–515.

Salonen J.T., Salonen R., Seppanen K., Rinta-Kukka S., Kukka M., Kopela H., Alfthan G., Kantola M. & Schalch W. (1991) Effect of antioxidant supplementation on platelet function: a randomised pair-matched, placebo-controlled, double-blind trial in men with low antioxidant status. *Am J Clin Nutr* **53**, 1222–9.

Schwartz P.L. & Rutherford I.M. (1981) The effect of tocopherol on high-density lipoprotein cholesterol. *Am J Clin Pathol* **76**, 843–4.

Sharman I.M., Down M.G. & Norgan N.G. (1976) The effects of vitamin E on physiological function and athletic performance of trained swimmers. *J Sports Med* **16**, 215–25.

Shute W.E., Shute E.V. & Vogelsang A. (1948) Vitamin E in angina pectoris. *Lancet* **1**, 301–2.

Stahelin H.B., Rosel F., Buess E. & Brubacher G. (1984) Cancer, vitamins, and plasma lipids: prospective Basel study. *J Natl Cancer Inst* **73**, 1463–8.

Spielberg S.P., Boxer L.A., Corash L.M. & Schulman J.D. (1979) Improved erythrocyte survival with high-dose vitamin E in chronic hemolyzing G6PD and glutathione synthetase deficiencies. *Ann Int Med* **90**, 53–4.

Stampfer M.J., Willett W., Castelli W.P., Taylor J.O., Fine J. & Hennekens C.H. (1983) Effect of vitamin E on lipids. *Am J Clin Pathol* **79**, 714–6.

Stampfer M.J., Jakubowski J.A., Faigel D., Vaillancourt R. & Deykin D. (1988) Vitamin E supplementation effect on human platelet function, arachidonic acid metabolism, and platelet prostacyclin levels. *Am J Clin Nutr* **47**, 700–6.

Steiner M. (1987) Effect of vitamin E on platelet function and thrombosis. *Agents Actions* **22**, 357–8.

Sundaram G.S., London R., Manimekalai S., Nair P.P. & Goldstein P. (1981) Alpha-tocopherol and serum lipoproteins. *Lipids* **16**, 223–7.

Wald N.J., Boreham J., Hayward J.L. & Bulbrook R.D. (1984) Plasma retinol, beta-carotene and vitamin E levels in relation to the future risk of breast cancer. *Br J Cancer* **49**, 321–4.

Wald N.J., Thompson S.G., Densem J.W., Boreham J. & Bailey A. (1987) Serum vitamin E and subsequent risk of cancer. *Br J Cancer* **56**, 69–72.

Willett W.C., Polk B.F., Underwood B.A., Stampfer M.J., Pressel S, Rossner B., Taylor J.O., Schneider K. & Hames C.G. (1984) Relation of serum vitamins A and E and carotenoids to the risk of cancer. *N Engl J Med* **310**, 662–6.

Williams H.T.G., Fenna D. & Macbeth R.A. (1971) Alpha tocopherol in the treatment of intermittent claudication. *Surg Gynecol Obstet* **132**, 662–6.

Chapter 55
Vitamin K

Description
Vitamin K is a fat-soluble vitamin.

Nomenclature
Vitamin K is a generic term for 2-methyl-1,4 naphthaquinone and all derivatives that exhibit qualitatively the biological activity of phytomenadione. The form of vitamin K present in foods is phytomenadione (vitamin K_1). The substances synthesized by bacteria are known as menaquinones (vitamin K_2). The parent compound of the vitamin K series is known as menadione (vitamin K_3); it is not a natural substance and is not used in humans. Menadiol sodium phosphate is a water-soluble derivative of menadione.

Human requirements
No Reference Nutrient Intake or Estimated Average Intake has been set, but a safe and adequate intake is for adults, 1 µg/kg daily; infants, 10 µg daily.
Some of the requirement for vitamin K is met by synthesis in the intestine.

Action
Vitamin K is an essential cofactor for the hepatic synthesis of proteins involved in the regulation of blood clotting. These are:

- prothrombin (factor II),
- factors VII, IX, X, and
- proteins C, S and Z.

Vitamin K is also required for the biosynthesis of some other proteins found in bone, plasma and kidney.

Dietary sources

Food Portion	Vitamin K content (µg)
Broccoli, boiled (100 g)	175
Brussels sprouts, boiled (100 g)	100
Cabbage, boiled (100 g)	125
Cauliflower, boiled (100 g)	150
Kale, boiled (100 g)	700
Lettuce (30 g)	45
Spinach, boiled (100 g)	400
Soya beans, cooked (100 g)	190
Meat–average, cooked (100 g)	50
Cheese (100 g)	50
Bread and cereals (100 g)	< 10 µg
Fruit (100 g)	< 10 µg

Excellent sources (> 100 µg/portion) (**bold**).

Metabolism

Absorption

Vitamin K is absorbed into the lymphatic system, predominantly in the upper part of the small intestine (jejunum and ileum), by a process which requires bile salts and pancreatic juice. The absorption of the different forms of vitamin K differs. Vitamin K_1 (phytomenadione) is absorbed by an active energy-dependent process from the proximal portion of the small intestine; menadione is absorbed by a passive non-carrier-mediated process from both the small and large intestines.

There is evidence that bacterially synthesized K can be a source of vitamin K for humans, although the availability of a sufficient concentration of bile salts for absorption is questionable (plasma levels of menaquinones suggest that some absorption occurs).

Distribution

Vitamin K is transported in the plasma and metabolized in the liver. Vitamin K_1 is concentrated and retained in the liver. Menadione is poorly retained by the liver but widely distributed in all other tissues.

Elimination

Vitamin K is eliminated partly in the bile (30–40%) and partly in the urine (15%).

Bioavailability

The effect of cooking and food processing on vitamin K has not been carefully studied, but vitamin K appears to be relatively stable.

Deficiency

Deficiency leads to a prolonged prothrombin time which can be corrected by vitamin K supplementation.

Uses

Vitamin K is not in common use as a dietary supplement. There is a medically recognized indication for infants (see Chapter 58).

Pregnancy and breast-feeding

No problems reported.

Adverse effects

Oral ingestion of natural forms of vitamin K is not associated with toxicity. A rare hypersensitivity reaction (occasionally results in death) has been reported after intravenous administration of phytomenadione (especially if rapid).

Interactions

Drugs

Antibiotics: may increase requirement for vitamin K.
Anti-coagulants: anticoagulant effect reduced by vitamin K. (Vitamin K is present in several tube feeds).
Cholestyramine or colestipol: may reduce intestinal absorption of vitamin K.
Liquid paraffin: may reduce intestinal absorption of vitamin K (avoid long-term use of liquid paraffin).
Sucralfate: may reduce intestinal absorption of vitamin K.

Nutrients

Vitamin A: under conditions of hypervitaminosis A hypothrombinaemia may occur; it can be corrected by administering vitamin K.
Vitamin E: large doses of vitamin E (1200 mg daily) increase the vitamin K requirement in patients taking anti-coagulants, but no confirmed effect in individuals not taking anti-coagulants.

Dose

Dietary supplements are unnecessary.

Chapter 56
Zinc

Description
Zinc is an essential trace mineral.

Human requirements

Dietary Reference Values (mg/d)

Age	RNI	EAR	LRNI
0–6 months	4.0	3.3	2.6
7 months–3 years	5.0	3.8	3.0
4–6 years	6.5	5.0	4.0
7–10 years	7.0	5.4	4.0
Males			
11–14 years	9.0	7.0	5.3
15–50+ years	9.5	7.3	5.5
Females			
11–14 years	9.0	7.0	5.3
15–50+ years	7.0	5.5	4.0
Pregnancy	7.0	5.5	4.0
Lactation			
0–4 months	13.0		
4+ months	9.5		

Reproduced and adapted with the permission of the Controller of Her Majesty's Stationery Office.

Intakes
In the UK the average adult diet provides: for men, 11.7 mg daily; for women, 8.7 mg.

Action
Zinc is an essential component of over 200 enzymes. It plays an important role in the metabolism of proteins, carbohydrates, lipids and nucleic acids and is involved in gene expression. Zinc is also crucial for maintaining the structure and integrity of cell membranes (loss of zinc results in an increased susceptibility to oxidative damage).

Dietary sources

Food portion	Zinc content (mg)
Breakfast cereals	
1 bowl All-Bran (45 g)	*3.0*
1 bowl Bran Flakes (45 g)	*1.5*
1 bowl Corn Flakes (30 g)	0.1
1 bowl Muesli (95 g)	*2.0*
2 pieces Shredded Wheat	1.0
2 Weetabix	1.0
Cereal products	
Bread, brown, 2 slices	0.7
white, 2 slices	0.4
wholemeal, 2 slices	1.3
1 chapati	0.7
Pasta, brown, boiled (150 g)	*1.5*
white, boiled (150 g)	0.7
Rice, brown, boiled (165 g)	1.0
white, boiled (165 g)	1.0
Milk and dairy products	
½ pint milk, whole, semi-skimmed or skimmed	1.0
1 pot yoghurt (150 g)	1.0
Cheese, Brie (50 g)	1.0
Camembert (50 g)	1.3
Cheddar (50 g)	1.1
Cheddar, reduced fat (50 g)	1.4
Cottage cheese (100 g)	0.5
Cream cheese (30 g)	0.2
Edam (50 g)	1.1
Feta (50 g)	0.4
Fromage Frais (100 g)	0.3
White cheese (50 g)	*1.5*
1 egg, size 2 (60 g)	0.8
Meat and fish	
Red meat, roast (85 g)	*4.0*
1 beef steak (155 g)	**7.0**
Minced beef, lean, stewed (100 g)	**6.0**
1 chicken leg (190 g)	*2.0*
Liver, lambs, cooked (90 g)	*4.0*
Kidney, lambs, cooked (75 g)	*3.0*
Fish	
Pilchards, canned (105 g)	*1.5*
Sardines, canned (70 g)	*2.0*
Crab (100 g)	**5.5**
1 dozen oysters	**78.7**

Food portion	Zinc content (mg)
Vegetables	
Green vegetables, average, boiled (100 g)	0.4
Potatoes, boiled (150 g)	0.5
1 small can baked beans (200 g)	1.0
Lentils, kidney beans or other pulses (105 g)	1.0
Dahl, chickpea (155 g)	*1.5*
lentil (155 g)	*1.5*
Soya beans, cooked (100 g)	1.0
Fruit	
8 dried apricots	0.2
4 figs	0.3
Half an avocado pear	0.3
1 banana	0.2
Blackberries (100 g)	0.2
Blackcurrants (100 g)	0.3
Nuts	
20 almonds	0.6
10 Brazil nuts	1.0
30 Hazelnuts	0.7
1 small bag peanuts (25 g)	1.0

Excellent sources (**bold**); good sources (*italics*).
Information derived from *The Composition of Foods*, 5th Edition (1991) is reproduced with the permission of The Royal Society of Chemistry and the Controller of Her Majesty's Stationery Office.

Metabolism

Absorption
Absorption occurs throughout the length of the small intestine, mostly in the jejunum, both by a carrier-mediated process and by diffusion.

Distribution
Zinc is transported in association with albumin, amino acids and a 2-macroglobulin. About 60% is stored in skeletal muscle and 30% in bone, with 4–6% in the skin. Highest concentrations are found in the iris, retina and choroid of the eye and in the prostate and spermatozoa.

Elimination
Elimination of zinc is mainly in the faeces; smaller amounts are excreted in the urine and via the skin.

Bioavailability
Absorption of zinc is enhanced by certain amino acids such as cysteine and histidine; the zinc content of meat, dairy produce and fish is therefore efficiently absorbed. Zinc from wholegrain cereals, including bran products, and also soy protein, is less available, due, in part, to the presence of phytate. The effect of non-starch polysaccharides (dietary fibre), tannic acid and caffeine is equivocal.

Deficiency

Clinical manifestations of severe zinc deficiency include:

- alopecia,
- diarrhoea,
- dermatitis,
- psychiatric disorder,
- weight loss,
- intercurrent infection (due to impaired immune function),
- hypogonadism in males, and
- poor ulcer healing.

Signs of mild to moderate deficiency include:

- growth retardation,
- male hypogonadism,
- poor appetite,
- rough skin,
- mental lethargy,
- delayed wound healing, and
- impaired taste acuity.

Maternal zinc deficiency before and during pregnancy may lead to intra-uterine growth retardation and congenital abnormalities in the foetus.

Uses

Anorexia nervosa

It has been suggested that zinc deficiency is involved in the aetiology of anorexia nervosa. Teenage girls who are restricting their food intake during the period of rapid growth may develop a state of zinc deficiency and anorexia nervosa. A daily supplement of 45 mg of zinc as zinc sulphate, has been reported to result in weight gain in 17 young female patients with long-standing anorexia nervosa (Safai-Kutti 1990). The weight gain continued over a 4-year follow-up period, and a multicentre clinical trial is now underway.

Wound healing

Zinc deficiency impairs wound repair by reducing the rate of epithelialization and cellular proliferation. Low zinc levels have been associated with poor wound healing and supplementation has promoted the healing process (Hallbrook & Lanner 1972; Thomas *et al*. 1988). Supplementation appears to be beneficial only in individuals who are zinc deficient (Weisman 1980).

In patients with gravitational ulcers, Husain (1969) reported a healing time of 32 days in patients who were given zinc supplements compared with 77 days in matched controls. However, this effect has not been reproduced in patients with venous ulcers (Phillips *et al*. 1972).

Miscellaneous

Zinc is of unproven value in the treatment of acne (Wiesmann *et al*. 1977) and the common cold.

Adverse effects

Signs of acute toxicity (doses > 200 mg daily) include gastro-intestinal pain, nausea, vomiting and diarrhoea. Prolonged exposure to doses > 50 mg daily may induce copper deficiency (marked by low serum copper and caeruloplasmin levels, microcytic anaemia and neutropenia) and iron deficiency. Doses > 150 mg daily may reduce serum HDL levels, depress immune function and cause gastric erosion.

Interactions

Drugs

4-quinotones: reduced absorption of 4-quinotones
Oral contraceptives: may reduce plasma zinc levels.
Penicillamine: reduced absorption of penicillamine.
Tetracyclines: reduced absorption of zinc and vice versa.

Nutrients

Copper: large doses of zinc may reduce absorption of copper.
Folic acid: may reduce zinc absorption (raises concern about pregnant women who are advised to take folic acid to reduce the risk of birth defects).
Iron: reduced absorption of oral iron and vice versa (raises concern about pregnant women who are often given iron; this may reduce zinc status and increase the risk of intra-uterine growth retardation and congenital abnormalities in the foetus).

Dose

Dietary supplements contain 5–50 mg (elemental zinc) per daily dose.
The zinc content of some commonly used zinc salts is as follows:

- zinc amino acid chelate (100 mg/g);
- zinc gluconate (130 mg/g);
- zinc orotate (170 mg/g); and
- zinc sulphate 227 mg/g).

References

Hallbrook T. & Lanner E. (1972) Serum zinc and healing of various leg ulcers. *Lancet* **2**, 780–2.
Husain S.L. (1969) Oral zinc supplementation in leg ulcers. *Lancet* **2**, 1069–71.
Phillips A., Davidson M. & Greaves M.W. (1972) Venous leg ulceration: evaluation of zinc treatment, serum zinc and rate of healing. *Clinical and Experimental Dermatology* **2**, 395–9.
Safai-Kutti S. (1990) Oral zinc supplementation in anorexia nervosa. *Acta Psychiatrica Scandinavica Supplementum* **361**, 82: 14–17.
Thomas A.J., Bunker V.W., Hinks L.J. *et al.* (1988) Energy, protein, zinc and copper status of 21 elderly inpatients: analysed dietary intake and biochemical indices. *Br J Nutr* **59**, 181–91.
Weisman K. (1980) Zinc metabolism in the skin. In: *Recent Advances in Dermatology.* (eds A. Rock & J.A. Savin), pp 109–29. Churchill Livingstone, Edinburgh.
Wiesmann K., Wadskov S., Sondergaard J. (1977) Oral zinc sulphate therapy in acne vulgaris. *Acta Dermatovenereologica* **57**, 357–60.

Chapter 57
Appendix 1: Product Index

There are over 3000 dietary supplement products available in the UK and space does not permit the provision of information for each one. Vitamin preparations which are prescription only medicines are not included.

Inclusion of a product in this list does not necessarily endorse its value or signify that the ingredients are efficacious or innocuous. Reference should be made to previous Chapters (3–56) for information on possible adverse effects, contra-indications, drug interactions and acceptable or controversial indications. It should also be noted that contents and strengths (where stated) are as described by the manufacturers.

Manufacturers' full names and addresses, telephone and facsimile numbers can be found in Chapter 59, Appendix 3.

Single ingredient products

Betacarotene
6 mg: Betacarotene capsules (Lamberts; Natures Best; Natures Own)
15 mg: Betacarotene capsules (Lamberts; Natural Flow; Natures Aid; Natures Best; Phoenix; Quest; Seven Seas; Solgar; Vitalia)
Betacarotene tablets (Larkhall)
Capseco capsules (Britannia)
FSC Beta Plus capsules (Health & Diet Food)
Healthcrafts Betacarotene capsules (Ferrosan Healthcare)
Pervita capsules (Lifeplan)

Bioflavonoids
250 mg: Pure-Fill Bioflavonoid capsules (Bio-Health)
300 mg: Bioflavonoids capsules (Lamberts; Natures Best)
500 mg: Cantassium Bioflavonoids Naturtabs (Larkhall)
Pure-Fill Bioflavonoid capsules (Bio-Health)

Biotin
200 µg: Biotin tablets (Natural Flow)
300 µg: Biotin tablets (Solgar)
500 µg: Biotin capsules (Lamberts; Natures Best); Biotin tablets (Larkhall)
800 µg: Health Aid tablets (Pharmadass)
1000 µg: Biotin tablets (Solgar)

Bonemeal
Available from Lane; Larkhall; Lifeplan; Solgar

Boron

3 mg: Borodol Naturtabs (Larkhall)
Boron 3 tablets (Lifeplan)
Boron Plus capsules (Lamberts; Natures Best)
Multi-chelated Boron capsules (Solgar)
Synergistic Boron capsules (Quest)

Brewer's Yeast

300 mg: Brewer's Yeast tablets (Gerard; Healthilife; Lifeplan; Natures Aid; Natures Own; Phillips Yeast; Phoenix); Yestamin tablets (English Grains)

500 mg: Brewer's Yeast tablets (Blackmores)
600 mg: Brewer's Yeast tablets (Solgar)

Calcium

Note: (Elemental calcium content per tablet or capsule is given in brackets when declared on product labels).

Non-proprietary products

Calcium Gluconate 600 mg tablets (53.4 mg)
Calcium Gluconate 1 g effervescent tablets (89 mg)
Calcium Lactate 300 mg tablets (39 mg)
Calcium with ergocalciferol tablets (97 mg)
Calcium Lactate 300 mg tablets (39 mg)
Calcium & ergocalciferol tablets (97 mg)

Proprietary products

Available from:

Bioceuticals:	Sea-Cal chewable tablets (500 mg)
Bio-Health:	Pure-Fill Extra Calcium capsules (167 mg)
Blackmores:	Bio Calcium tablets
Cedar Health:	Minalka tablets (22 mg)
	Porosis D tablets (115 mg)
English Grains:	Calcia tablets (300 mg)
	Calcia Chewable tablets (800 mg)
Health & Diet:	FSC Calcium plus A & D tablets (250 mg)
	FSC Super Cal/Mag tablets (500 mg)
Ferrosan	Healthcrafts Aminochel Calcium tablets (75 mg)
Healthcare:	Chewable Calcium tablets (500 mg)
	Super Calcium Plus tablets (42 mg)
Illingworth:	Healthwise Super Osteocal tablets (250 mg)
	Healthwise Calcium with Vitamins A & D tablets (250 mg)
Lamberts:	Calcium Amino Acid Chelate capsules (125 mg)
	Calcium Citrate capsules
	Cal/Mag Balance capsules (33 mg)
	Calcium Orotate tablets (51 mg)
	Calcium Extra tablets (500 mg)
	Calcium/Magnesium Orotates capsules (30 mg)

	Cal/Mag/Zinc Orotates capsules (25 mg)
	Calcium 500 Magnesium 250 Amino Acid Chelate tablets (500 mg)
Lane:	Calcium tablets (150 mg)
	Earthlore Calcium with Magnesium tablets
Larkhall:	B13 Calcium Naturtabs (500 mg)
	B13 Cal. Dri-fil Naturtabs
	Calcimega 500 Naturtabs (500 mg)
Lifeplan:	Caltabs tablets (500 mg)
	Chewable Calcium tablets (500 mg)
3M:	Titralac tablets (170 mg)
Natural Flow:	Calcium Special Delivery tablets (250 mg)
	Calcium/Magnesium tablets
	Milk Free Calcium tablets
Natures Aid:	Good Health Chewable Calcium tablets (500 mg)
Natures Best:	Calcium Citrate capsules (100 mg)
	Calcium Phosphate tablets (150 mg)
	Calcium/Magnesium tablets (500 mg)
	Osteo-Balance capsules (33 mg)
Natures Own:	Calcium & Magnesium Carbonates tablets (500 mg)
	Calcium Orotate 500 mg tablets (85 mg)
	Food State Calcium tablets (30 mg)
	Food State Calcium and Vitamin D tablets (300 mg)
Pharma-Nord:	Bio-Calcium+D3 tablets (164 mg)
Pharmadass:	Strong Calcium tablets (500 mg)
Phoenix:	Equal Ratio Cal–Mag tablets (100 mg)
	Equal Ratio High Potency Cal–Mag Plus tablets (250 mg)
Power:	Calcium 400 tablets (400 mg)
	Tri Calc tablets
Procter & Gamble:	Cacit tablets (500 mg)
Renacare:	Calcium–500 tablets (500 mg)
Shire:	Calcichew tablets (500 mg)
	Calcichew Forte tablets (1 g)
	Calcichew D3 tablets (500 mg)
	Calcidrink sachets (1 g)
	Citrical sachets (500 mg)
Quest:	Balanced Ratio Cal–Mag tablets (100 mg)
Seven Seas:	Berries Calcium with Vitamin D (500 mg)
Solgar:	Calci-Chews wafers (500 mg)
	Calcium "600" tablets (600 mg)
	Calcium Citrate with D tablets (250 mg)
	Calcium Magnesium tablets (250 mg)
	Calcium Magnesium Citrate tablets (200 mg)
	Chelated Calcium tablets (833 mg)
Vitabiotics:	Osteocare tablets (300 mg)

Carnitine

250 mg:	L-Carnitine tablets (Lamberts & Larkhall)
500 mg:	L-Carnitine tablets (Solgar)

Choline & Inositol

Available from: Health Plus; Lamberts; Larkhall; Natural Flow; Natures Best; Pharmadass; Phoenix; Solgar

Chromium

60 μg: Food State GTF tablets (Natures Own)
100 μg: GTF Chromium capsules (Lamberts; Natures Best) GTF chromium tablets (Solgar)
200 μg: Chromium Amino Acid Chelate capsules (Lamberts)
Chromium capsules (Phoenix)
Chromium tablets (Natural Flow; Solgar; Wassen)
FSC ChromeActive capsules (Health & Diet)

Co-enzyme Q

10 mg: Co-enzyme Q10 capsules (Healthilife; Lamberts; Lifeplan; Natural Flow)
15 mg: Co-enzyme Q10 capsules (Phoenix; Quest)
20 mg: Health Aid capsules (Pharmadass)
30 mg: Bio-Quinone Q10 (Pharma Nord) Co-enzyme Q10 capsules (Natures Aid; Quest)
Maxi CoQ-10 capsules (Solgar) 60 mg: CoQ-60 capsules (Solgar)

Copper

2.5 mg: Chelated Copper tablets (Solgar)
3 mg: Copper tablets (Natural Flow)
50 mg: B13 Copper Naturtabs

Dolomite

Available from: Gerard; Ferrosan Healthcare; Health & Diet; Health Plus; Illingworth; Lane; Lamberts; Larkhall; Natural Flow; Natures Aid; Natures Best; Natures Own; Power, Solgar

Evening Primrose Oil

Note: Evening primrose oil normally contains 8–10% of gamma-linolenic acid (GLA); starflower oil (borage oil) is added to some products to increase the GLA content. The strengths listed relate to the content of evening primrose oil, not the GLA content.

250 mg: Evening Primrose Oil capsules (Healthilife; Lamberts; Natures Best; Natures Own; Reevecrest)
Efamol capsules (Efamol)
EPOC capsules (Evening Primrose Oil)
FSC Evening Primrose Oil capsules (Health & Diet)
Glanolin capsules (Lane)
Healthcrafts Evening Primrose Oil capsules (Ferrosan Healthcare)
Healthwise Evening Primrose Oil capsules (Illingworth)
Seven Seas Berries Evening Primrose Oil (Seven Seas)
Super Galanol capsules (Lifeplan)
500 mg: Evening Primrose Oil capsules (Bio-Health; Brithealth; Gerard; Healthilife; Lamberts; Lane; Natural Flow; Natures Aid; Natures

Best; Natures Own; Neutraceuticals; Pharmadass; Quest; Solgar; Unichem; Vitalia)
BritEpo Evening Primrose Oil capsules (Brithealth)
Efamol capsules (Efamol)
EPOC capsules (Evening Primrose Oil)
Evoprim capsules (Bioceuticals)
FSC Evening Primrose Oil capsules (Health & Diet)
Galanol GLX capsules (Lifeplan)
Galanol Gold capsules (Lifeplan)
Glanolin capsules (Lane)
Good Health Evening Primrose Oil capsules (Natures Aid)
Healthcrafts Evening Primrose Oil capsules (Ferrosan Healthcare)
Healthwise Evening Primrose Oil capsules (Illingworth)
Lantier Evening Primrose Oil capsules (Myplan)
Sanatogen Evening Primrose Oil capsules (Roche)
Seven Seas High Strength Super Evening Primrose Oil capsules (Seven Seas)
Super GLA capsules (Larkhall)

1000 mg: Evening Primrose Oil capsules (Brithealth; Healthilife; Lamberts; Natural Flow; Natures Aid; Natures Best; Neutraceuticals; Pharmadass; Quest; Unichem; Vitalia)
EPOC capsules (Evening Primrose Oil)
Evoprim capsules (Bioceuticals)
FSC Evening Primrose Oil capsules (Health & Diet)
Galanol GLX capsules (Lifeplan)
Galanol Gold capsules (Lifeplan)
Healthcrafts Evening Primrose Oil capsules (Ferrosan Healthcare)
Healthwise Evening Primrose Oil capsules (Illingworth)
Seven Seas Premium Strength Super Evening Primrose Oil capsules (Seven Seas)
Super GLA capsules (Larkhall).

Fish Oil

Note: Contents of eicosapentaenoic acid (EPA) and docosohexaenoic acid (DHA) are stated in brackets (in the order EPA/DHA) where declared on product labels.
Available from:

Bio-Health: Super Cod Liver Oil Two-A-Day capsules (50 mg/34 mg)
Brithealth: Capseco Cod Liver Oil capsules
Capseco Marine Fish Oil capsules
Pure Cod Liver Oil One-a-day Capsules
Pure Omega Fish Oil Capsules (700 mg total EPA/DHA)
Callanish: Marine with Vitamin E capsules
Golden Health Cod Liver Oil capsules
Ferrosan Healthcare: Healthcrafts Cod Liver Oil capsules
Healthcrafts Compleat Cod Liver Oil capsules
Healthcrafts EPA Forte capsules (320 mg/210 mg)
Healthcrafts Super Halibut Liver Oil capsules
Gerard: Cod Liver Oil capsules

	Halibut Liver Oil capsules
Health & Diet:	FSC Cod Liver Oil capsules
	FSC Hi-Potency Cod Liver Oil capsules
	FSC Super Cod Liver Oil capsules
	Foil Fish Oil capsules
Healthilife:	Pure Cod Liver Oil capsules
	Pure Cod Liver Oil One-a-Day capsules
	Pure Cod Liver Oil liquid
	Cod Liver Oil with Evening Primrose Oil liquid
	High Strength Cod Liver Oil with EPA & DHA capsules
	Cod Liver Oil with Multivitamins capsules
	Halibut Liver Oil capsules
	Fish Oil Complex One-a-Day capsules (70 mg/26 mg)
	Fish Oil & Odourless Garlic One-a-Day capsules
Health Plus:	E.P.A capsules (180 mg/120 mg)
Illingworth:	Healthwise Cod Liver Oil capsules
	Cod Liver Oil One-a-Day With Vitamins A, D & E capsules
	Cod Liver Oil One-a-Day High Strength capsules
	Fish Oil Omega 3 capsules (180 mg/120 mg)
	Halibut Liver Oil capsules
Lamberts:	Cod Liver Oil capsules
	EPA Marine Lipid Concentrate capsules (180 mg/ 120 mg)
	High Potency EPA capsules (310 mg/210 mg)
Lane:	Fish Factor Capsules
	Halibut Liver Oil A & D capsules
	Lanepa Fish Oil capsules (180 mg/120 mg)
	Lanepa Fish Oil liquid (830 mg/550 mg in 5 ml)
Larkhall:	Cod Liver Oil Capsules
	Halibut Liver Oil capsules
	Mega Fish Oil capsules (500 mg total EPA/DHA)
Lifeplan:	Cod Liver Oil capsules
	Cod Liver Oil & Garlic O.A.D. 502 mg capsules
	Flowmega EPA/DHA capsules (80 mg/45 mg)
	Marinepa capsules
Natural Care:	Cod Liver Oil capsules
	Fish Oil capsules
Natural Flow:	EPA Forte Complex capsules
	Fish Oil Vitamin A and D capsules
Natures Aid:	Cod Liver Oil capsules
	Salmon Oil capsules
Natures Best:	High Potency EPA capsules (320 mg/210 mg)
	EPA 180 capsules (180 mg/120 mg)
	Complete Cod Liver Oil capsules
	Cod Liver Oil capsules
Natures Own:	Cod Liver Oil capsules
	Halibut Liver Oil capsules
Novex Pharma:	Maxepa capsules (180 mg/120 mg)
	Maxepa emulsion (900 mg/600 mg in 10 ml)

	Maxepa liquid (900 mg/600 mg in 10 ml)
Pharma-Nord:	Bio-Marine capsules (175 mg/ 125 mg)
Pharmadass:	Mega Cod Liver Oil capsules (114 mg/91 mg)

Cod Liver Oil with Evening Primrose Oil capsules (50 mg/ 40 mg)

Cod Liver Oil with Odourless Garlic Oil capsules (15 mg/ 13 mg)

Cod Liver Oil with Multivitamins and Minerals capsules

Halibut Liver Oil capsules

Marine Fish Oils capsules (180 mg/120 mg)

EPA 1000 capsules (310 mg/210 mg)

Phoenix: EPA 1000 Fish Lipid Concentrate capsules (135 mg/90 mg)

Power: Cod Liver Oil capsules

Cod Liver Oil One-a-Day capsules

Halibut Liver Oil capsules

Hi EPA capsules

Icelandic Gold Cod Liver Oil liquid

Mini Cod capsules

Salmon Oil capsules

Quest: Gamma EPA capsules (180 mg/120 mg)

Pure Cod Liver Oil capsules: standard strength (20 mg/20 mg); high strength (114/75 mg)

Roche: Sanatogen Cod Liver Oil (828 mg/828 mg in 10 ml)

Sanatogen Cod Liver Oil capsules (24 mg/21 mg)

Sanatogen Cod Liver Oil plus Multivitamins capsules (36 mg/ 24 mg)

Sanatogen Pure Fish Oils capsules (90 mg/60 mg)

Pulse Fish Oils capsules (70 mg/45 mg)

Pulse High Strength Fish Oils capsules (200 mg/60.8 mg)

Pulse High Strength liquid (900 mg/300 mg in 5 ml)

Seven Seas: Pure Cod Liver Oil liquid (828 mg/736 mg in 10 ml)

Pure Cod Liver Oil capsules (26 mg/24 mg)

Pure Cod Liver Oil One-A-Day capsules

Pure Cod Liver Oil High Strength One-A-Day capsules (82.8 mg/73.6 mg)

High Strength Pure Cod Liver Oil (1242 mg/1102 mg in 10 ml)

Pure Cod Liver Oil with Evening Primrose Oil capsules (52.5 mg/46.7 mg)

Lemon Flavour Pure Cod Liver Oil Spoonful liquid (788 mg/ 700 mg in 10 ml)

Lemon Flavour Pure Cod Liver Oil with EPO liquid (744 mg/ 661 mg in 10 ml)

Orange Syrup and Cod Liver Oil liquid (252 mg/224 mg in 10 ml)

Pure Fish Oils capsules

Pure Fish Oils and Kelp capsules (31.5 mg/20.3 mg)

Solgar: Cod Liver Oil Softgels

One-a-Day EPA/GLA Softgels (180 mg/120 mg)

Super EPA Softgels (230 mg/153 mg)

	Omega-3 '700' Softgels (400 mg/300 mg)
Unichem:	Cod Liver Oil capsules
Vitalia:	Cod Liver Oil Super capsules
	Salmon Oil EPA Rich capsules
Wassen:	Omega-3 Concentrated Fish Oil capsules (105 mg total EPA/DHA)

Fluoride

En-De-Kay (Stafford Miller)	Fluodrops
	Fluotabs 2–4 years
	Fluotabs 4+ years
Fluor-a-day (Dental Health)	Tablets: 1.1 mg, 2.2 mg
FluoriGard (Colgate-Palmolive)	Drops
	Tablets: 0.5 mg, 1 mg
Oral-B Fluoride (Oral-B)	Tablets: 0.5 mg, 1 mg

Folic Acid

400 µg:	Folic acid capsules (Natures Best)
	Folic acid tablets (Lamberts; Quest; Solgar)
	Cantassium Folic acid tablets (Larkhall)
	FSC Folic Acid tablets (Health & Diet)
	Folic 400 tablets (Health Plus)
	Good Health Folic Acid tablets (Natures Aid)
	Health Aid Folic Acid tablets (Pharmadass)
	Preconceive tablets (Lane)
	Seven Seas Folic Plus capsules (Seven Seas)
500 µg:	Cantassium Folic acid Naturtabs (Larkhall)
800 µg:	Folic acid tablets (Natural Flow; Solgar)
1000 µg:	Cantassium Folic acid Naturtabs (Larkhall)
5000 µg:	Folic acid tablets (Lamberts)

Garlic

Biol-Health	
Garlic capsules	Dried garlic 250 mg
Healthilife	
Mega garlic pearles	Garlic oil 5 mg
Odourless garlic pearles	Garlic powder 0.66 mg
One a day Odourless garlic pearles	Garlic powder 2 mg
Golden garlic Pearls	Garlic oil 0.66 mg
Healthwise (Illingworth)	
Garlic oil capsules	Garlic concentrate 1.05 mg
Odourless garlic	Fresh garlic equivalance 1000 mg
Japanese garlic	Garlic extract 40 mg
Health Aid (Pharmadass)	
Garlic oil odourless	Garlic oil 2 mg
Health Plus	
Premier Garlic	Garlic concentrate 500 mg
Heath & Heather	
(Ferrosan Healthcare)	
Odourless Garlic Perles	Garlic powder 0.66 mg

One a day Odourless Garlic Perles	Garlic powder 2 mg
Hofels (Seven Seas)	
Original Garlic Pearles	Garlic oil 0.66 mg
One a day Garlic Pearles	Garlic oil 2 mg
Kwai (Lichtwer Pharma)	Dried garlic 100 mg
Kyolic (Quest)	
Kyolic 100	Garlic extract 300 mg
Kyolic 102	Garlic extract 350 mg
Kyolic 404	Garlic extract 100 mg
Lamberts	
Pure-Gar	Garlic powder 500 mg
Garlic oil capsules	Garlic oil 2 mg
Lusty (Lane)	
Garlic Perles	Garlic oil 0.66 mg
Natural Flow	
Garlite	Dried garlic 500 mg
Natures Aid	
Odourless garlic pearls	Garlic powder 2 mg
Natures Own	
Garlic oil	Garlic oil 0.972 mg
Pharma-Nord	
Bio-Garlic	Dried garlic 300 mg
Sanatogen (Roche)	
Garlic perles	Garlic oil 2 mg
Seven Seas	
Garlic oil perles	Garlic oil 2 mg

Germanium
Available from Larkhall

Ginkgo Biloba
Available from: Ferrosan Healthcare (Idoloba); Health Dynamics (Ginkgo Forte); Lamberts; Pharma-Nord (Bio-Biloba)

Ginseng
Available from: Biocare; Bio-Health; Blackmores; Callanish; English Grains (Red Kooga range); Ferrosan Healthcare (Healthcrafts range); Health & Diet (FSC range); Healthilife; Health World; IL HWA Ginseng; Illingworth; Jessup; Larkhall; Lifeplan; Man Shuen Hong; Natural Flow; Natures Aid; Natures Best; Natures Own; Pharmadass; Phoenix; Power; Quest; Reevecrest; Roche (Sanatogen range); Seven Seas; Solgar; Vitalife; Weider (Schiff range)

Green Lipped Mussel
Available from: Ferrosan Healthcare (Seatone range); Illingworth; Larkhall; Natures Best; Phoenix; Power

Guarana
Available from: Bioceuticals; Lifeplan; Natures Best; Power; Rio Amazon

Iodine
100 mg: Bioiodine tablets (Bioceuticals)

Iron
    Note: Elemental iron content per capsule or tablet is given in brackets.

Non-proprietary products
    Ferrous Sulphate 200 mg tablets (65 mg)
    Ferrous Gluconate 300 mg tablets (35 mg)

Proprietary products
    Available from:

Abbott:	Ferrograd Filmtabs (105 mg)
	Ferrograd C Filmtabs (105 mg)
	Ferrograd Folic Filmtabs (105 mg)
ASTA Medica:	Ferrocontin Continus tablets (100 mg)
	Ferrocontin Folic Continus tablets (105 mg)
Bio-Health:	Pure-Fill Extra Iron capsules (20 mg)
Ciba:	Slow Fe tablets (50 mg)
	Slow Fe Folic tablets (50 mg)
Consolidated:	Ferrocap capsules (110 mg)
	Ferrocap F capsules (110 mg)
Evans:	Fefol spansules (47 mg)
	Fefol-vit spansules (47 mg)
	Fefol-Z spansules (47 mg)
	Feospan spansules (47 mg)
	Fersaday tablets (100 mg)
	Fesovit-Z spansules (47 mg)
	Pregaday tablets (100 mg)
Ferrosan Healthcare:	Healthcrafts Aminochel Iron tablets (8 mg)
	Iron Plus tablets (6.2 mg)
Forley:	Fersamal syrup (45 mg/5 ml)
	Fersamal tablets (65 mg)
Galen:	Galfer capsules (100 mg)
	Galfer syrup (45 mg/5 ml)
	Galfer FA capsules (100 mg)
	Givitol capsules (100 mg)
Gerard:	Iron Complex tablets
Goldshield:	Pregnavite Forte F tablets (25.2 mg)
Health & Diet:	FSC Blackstrap Molasses Iron capsules
Healthilife:	Amino Acid Chelated Iron capsules (12 mg)
Illingworth:	Healthwise Iron Aid Plus tablets
Lamberts:	Iron Amino Acid Chelate tablets (24 mg)
Lane:	Iron capsules (20 mg)
	Earthlore Iron tablets
Larkhall:	Foresight Iron tablets (7 mg)
	Iron Formula tablets (6 mg)
	B13 Iron Naturtabs (50 mg)

Lifeplan:	Iron Formula with Vitamins B & C tablets
	Quadiron tablets
Link:	Plesmet syrup (25 mg/5 ml)
Natural Flow:	Iron tablets (40 mg)
Natures Best:	Iron Amino Acid Chelate tablets (24 mg)
Natures Own:	Food State Iron and Molybdenum tablets (5 mg)
Pharmadass:	Health Aid Strong Iron Formula tablets (5 mg)
Phoenix:	Bio-Enhanced Iron capsules (25 mg)
Quest:	Synergistic Iron capsules (25 mg)
RP Drugs:	Lexpec with Iron-M syrup (80 mg/5 ml)
Rybar:	Folex-350 tablets (100 mg)
Seven Seas:	Berries Iron with Vitamin C capsules (4 mg)
Sinclair:	Meterfolic tablets (100 mg)
SmithKline	
Beecham:	Iron Jelloids capsules (20 mg)
Solgar:	Chelated Iron tablets (30 mg)
	Gentle Iron Vegicaps (30 mg)
Tillomed:	Niferex elixir (100 mg/5 ml)
	Niferex-150 capsules (150 mg)
Vitalia:	Iron Formula + Folic Acid tablets

Kelp

Available from: Bio-Health; Blackmores; Ferrosan Healthcare (Healthcrafts range); Health & Diet (FSC range); Healthilife; Larkhall; Lifeplan; Natural Flow; Natures Aid; Natures Best; Natures Own; Pharmadass; Phoenix; Power; Solgar.

Lactobacillus

Available from: Bioceuticals; Blackmores; Health & Diet (FSC range); Illingworth (Healthwise range); Lamberts; Larkhall; Lifeplan; Myplan (Lactaid range); Natural Flow; Natures Best; Natures Own; Pharmadass; Phoenix; Power; Quest; Solgar.

Lecithin

Available from: Bioceuticals; Blackmores; Ferrosan Healthcare (Healthcrafts range); Gerard; Healthilife; Health Plus; Illingworth (Healthwise range); Lamberts; Lane; Larkhall; Lifeplan; Natural Flow; Natures Aid; Natures Best; Pharmadass; Phoenix; Power; Seven Seas; Solgar; Vitalia; Vitalife.

Magnesium

30 mg:	Food State Magnesium tablets (Natures Own)
50 mg:	Healthcrafts Aminochel Magnesium tablets (Ferrosan Healthcare)
60 mg:	Magnesium Formula and Calcium tablets (Vitalia)
100 mg:	Chelated Magnesium tablets (Solgar)
125 mg:	Magnesium Amino Acid Chelate tablets (Lamberts)
150 mg:	Bio-Enhanced Magnesium tablets (Phoenix)
	Synergistic Magnesium tablets (Quest)
	Time Release Magnesium tablets (Natures Best)
200 mg:	Magnesium Amino Acid Chelate tablets (Lamberts; Natures Best)

	Magnesium Citrate tablets (Solgar)
	Magnesium tablets (Natural Flow)
400 mg:	Magnesium Complex capsules (Lamberts)
	Magnesium + B6 tablets (Solgar)
500 mg:	B13 Magnesium Naturtabs (Larkhall)

Manganese
5 mg:	Manganese capsules (Lamberts; Natures Best)
20 mg:	Food State Manganese (Natures Own)
50 mg:	Bio-Enhanced Manganese capsules (Phoenix)
	Chelated Manganese tablets (Solgar)
	Manganese Amino Acid Chelate capsules (Lamberts)
	Manganese 50 mg tablets (Natural Flow)

Molybdenum
150 µg:	Chelated Molybdenum tablets (Solgar)

Niacin
100 mg:	Niacin tablets (Solgar)
	Nicotinamide capsules (Lamberts; Natures Best)
	Nicotinic acid capsules (Lamberts)
	Nicotinic acid tablets (Natural Flow)
	Cantassium Nicotinamide Naturtabs (Larkhall)
	Cantassium Nicotinic acid Naturtabs (Larkhall)
250 mg:	Niacin tablets (Blackmores; Natures Own)
500 mg:	Niacin capsules (Solgar)
	Niacin tablets (Phoenix)
	Niacinamide tablets (Phoenix)
	Nicotinamide capsules (Lamberts)
	Nicotinamide tablets (Natural Flow)
	Cantassium Nicotinamide Naturtabs (Larkhall)
	Cantassium Nicotinic acid Naturtabs (Larkhall)
	FSC Niacinamide tablets (Health & Diet)
	No-flush Niacin capsules (Solgar)
	Sustaniacin Naturtabs (Larkhall)
1000 mg:	Cantassium Nicotinamide Naturtabs (Larkhall)
	Cantassium Nicotinic acid Naturtabs (Larkhall)

Pangamic Acid
Available from: Lamberts; Larkhall; Natures Best; Natures Own; Phoenix

Pantothenic Acid
50 mg:	Cantopal Naturtabs (Larkhall)
100 mg:	Pantothenic acid capsules (Lamberts; Natures Best)
	Pantothenic acid tablets (Blackmores; Healthilife; Phoenix)
120 mg:	Pantothenic acid tablets (Gerard)
200 mg:	Pantothenic acid (Vitalife)
250 mg:	Pantothenic acid capsules (Quest)
	Pantothenic acid tablets (Lifeplan; Natures Own)
500 mg:	Pantothenic acid tablets (Lamberts; Natural Flow; Power)

Biovit–B5 tablets (Bioceuticals)
Cantopal Naturtabs (Larkhall)
FSC Pantothenic acid tablets (Health & Diet)
Healthwise Pantothenic acid tablets (Illingworth)
550 mg: Pantothenic acid capsules (Solgar)
750 mg: Health Aid Pantothenic acid tablets (Pharmadass)
1000 mg: Cantopal Naturtabs (Larkhall)

Para-amino benzoic acid

Available from: Bioceuticals; Lamberts; Larkhall; Natural Flow; Phoenix; Quest; Solgar

Potassium

Available in strengths of 100–200 mg from: Lamberts; Larkhall; Natural Flow; Natures Best; Natures Own; Phoenix; Power; Solgar.

Riboflavine

10 mg: Riboflavine capsules (Healthilife)
25 mg: Cantassium Riboflavine Naturtabs (Larkhall)
50 mg: Riboflavine capsules (Lamberts)
Riboflavine tablets (Blackmores; Natures Best)
100 mg: Riboflavine capsules (Phoenix; Solgar)
Riboflavine tablets (Natural Flow; Phoenix)

Royal Jelly

Available from: Bioceuticals (Biobees range); Brithealth (Royalgel range); Ferrosan Healthcare (Healthcrafts range); Health & Diet (FSC range); Healthilife; Health World; Illingworth (Healthwise range); Lamberts; Larkhall; Lifeplan; Natural Flow; Natures Aid; Natures Best; Pharmadass; Phoenix; Power; Quest; Reevecrest; Regina (Royal range); Seven Seas; Unichem; Vitalia; Vitalife; Weider (Schiff range).

Selenium

25 µg: Seven Seas Selenium with vitamin E capsules
50 µg: Selenium tablets (Health Plus; Lamberts; Natural Flow; Natures Best)
Seleno 6 tablets (Solgar)
100 µg: Selenium tablets (Lifeplan)
Food State Selenium tablets (Natures Own)
Seleno 6 tablets (Solgar)
Selenium ACE tablets (Wassen)
200 µg: Selenium capsules (Lamberts; Natures Best)
Bio-Enhanced Selenium capsules (Phoenix)
Food State Selenium tablets (Natures Own)
Seleno 6 tablets (Solgar)
Super Selenium 200 µg tablets (Natural Flow)
Synergistic Selenium capsules (Quest)

Silicon

Available from: Lamberts; Larkhall; Natures Best; Power

Spirulina
Available from: Bioceuticals; Lamberts; Lane; Larkhall; Lifestream; Natures Best; Phoenix

Starflower Oil
250 mg: Starflower oil capsules (Roche)
500 mg: Starflower oil capsules (Healthilife; Roche)
Sanatogen Starflower oil capsules (Roche)
1000 mg: Starflower oil capsules (Healthilife)

Superoxide dismutase
Available from: Larkhall; Lifeplan; Solgar

Thiamine
25 mg: Thiamine capsules (Healthilife)
Benerva tablets (Roche)
50 mg: Benerva tablets (Roche)
100 mg: Thiamine capsules (Lamberts; Phoenix; Solgar)
Thiamine tablets (Blackmores; Natures Best; Phoenix)
Thiamine Naturtabs (Larkhall)
Benerva tablets (Roche)
Healthwise Thiamine tablets (Illingworth)
250 mg: Thiamine Naturtabs (Larkhall)
300 mg: Thiamine tablets (Natural Flow)
Benerva tablets (Roche)
500 mg: Thiamine tablets (Solgar)

Vitamin A
2500 units: Vitamin A capsules (Healthilife)
FSC Vitamin A capsules (Health & Diet)
Healthcrafts Compleat Vitamin A tablets (Ferrosan Healthcare)
5000 units: Vitamin A tablets (Vitalia)
7500 units: Vitamin A capsules (Lamberts)
Vitamin A Softgels (Solgar)
Healthcrafts Super Vitamin A capsules (Ferrosan Healthcare)
10 000 units: Vitamin A capsules (Phoenix)
Vitamin A tablets (Blackmores)
25 000 units: Vitamin A capsules (Lamberts)
Vitamin A tablets (Natural Flow; Phoenix)
Cantassium Vitamin A capsules (Larkhall)

Vitamin B$_6$
10 mg: Vitamin B$_6$ capsules (Healthilife)
Vitamin B$_6$ tablets (Lane)
20 mg: Vitamin B$_6$ tablets (Vitalife)
Benadon tablets (Roche)
25 mg: Vitamin B$_6$ tablets (Lifeplan)
Healthcrafts Vitamin B$_6$ tablets (Ferrosan Healthcare)
40 mg: Seven Seas Super Vitamin B$_6$ capsules
50 mg: Vitamin B$_6$ tablets (Healthilife; Lamberts; Lifeplan; Natures Best;

Natures Own; Pharmadass; Quest; Vitalia; Vitalife)
Cantassium Vitamin B_6 Naturtabs (Larkhall)
FSC Vitamin B_6 tablets (Health & Diet Food)
Good Health Vitamin B_6 tablets (Natures Aid)
Sanatogen Vitamin B_6 tablets (Roche)

100 mg: Vitamin B_6 capsules (Lamberts; Natures Best; Solgar; Vitalife)
Vitamin B_6 tablets (Blackmores; Healthilife; Lane; Lifeplan; Natural
Flow; Natures Aid; Natures Own; Pharmadass; Power; Reevecrest)
Biovite–B6 tablets (Bioceuticals)
Cantassium Vitamin B_6 Naturtabs (Larkhall)
Complement Continus tablets (Napp)
FSC Vitamin B_6 tablets (Health & Diet)
Healthwise Vitamin B_6 tablets (Illingworth)

250 mg: Vitamin B_6 capsules (Solgar)
Vitamin B_6 tablets (Lamberts; Power)
Cantassium Vitamin B_6 Naturtabs
Naturetime Vitamin B_6 tablets (Blackmores)

Vitamin B_{12}
10 μg: Vitamin B_{12} capsules (Healthilife)
25 μg: Vitamin B_{12} tablets (Lifeplan)
50 μg: Vitamin B_{12} tablets (Solgar)
Cantassium Vitamin B_{12} Naturtabs (Larkhall)
Cytacon tablets (Evans)
100 μg: Vitamin B_{12} capsules (Lamberts; Natures Best)
Vitamin B_{12} tablets (Blackmores; Healthilife; Phoenix)
Healthwise Vitamin B_{12} tablets (Illingworth)
250 μg: Vitamin B_{12} tablets (Natural Flow)
500 μg: Vitamin B_{12} tablets (Power; Quest)
Biovit–B12 tablets (Bioceuticals)
1000 μg: Vitamin B_{12} capsules (Lamberts)
Vitamin B_{12} Lozenges
Vitamin B_{12} nuggets (Solgar)
Vitamin B_{12} tablets (Pharmadass)
Cantassium Vitamin B_{12} Naturtabs (Larkhall)

Vitamin C
20 mg: Redoxon tablets (Roche)
30 mg: Sanatogen Vitamin C tablets (Roche)
50 mg: Redoxon tablets (Roche)
75 mg: Vitamin C tablets (Unichem)
Biovit–C Vitamin tablets (Pharma-Nord)
90 mg: Good Health Vitamin C tablets (Natures Aid)
100 mg: Vitamin C caplets (Bioceuticals)
Vitamin C capsules (Gerard; Solgar)
Vitamin C tablets (Healthilife; Lamberts)
Flavorola-C tablets (Lane)
Tasty-C tablets (Natures Best)
200 mg: Vitamin C tablets (Healthilife; Lane; Natures Aid)
Redoxon tablets (Roche)

	Seven Seas Vitamin C Plus capsules (Seven Seas)
250 mg:	FSC Vitamin C tablets (Health & Diet)
	Food State Vitamin C tablets (Natures Own)
	Redoxon Chewable Vitamin C tablets (Roche)
300 mg:	Vitamin C capsules (Solgar)
	Vitamin C tablets (Lifeplan; Quest; Vitalife)
500 mg:	Vitamin C tablets (Healthilife; Illingworth; Lamberts; Lifeplan; Natures Aid; Natures Own; Phoenix; Power; Quest; Reevecrest; Roche; Solgar; Vitalife)
	Acerola Plus tablets (Natures Best)
	Bio–C tablets (Blackmores; Phoenix)
	C Buffered Chewable tablets (Vitalia)
	C Super tablets (Vitalia)
	C Time Release tablets (Vitalia)
	Cantassium Vitamin C Naturtabs (Larkhall)
	Earthlore Top–C tablets (Lane)
	Ester–C tablets (Lamberts; Natures Best)
	Ester–C vegicaps (Solgar)
	FSC Vitamin C tablets (Health & Diet)
	Gentle C tablets (Natures Best)
	Gentle Vitamin C tablets (Lamberts)
	Pure-Fill Vitamin C capsules (Bio-Health)
	Schiff Vitamin C tablets (Weider)
	Seven Seas Berries High Vitamin C capsules (Seven Seas)
	Super C tablets (Phoenix)
	Super Flavorola C tablets (Lifeplan)
	Ultra Vitamin C Complex capsules (Lamberts)
	Vital C capsules (Vitalife)
750 mg:	Bio–C Vitamin tablets (Pharma-Nord)
1000 mg:	Vitamin C tablets (Brithealth; Healthilife; Illingworth; Lamberts; Lifeplan; Natures Aid; Natures Best; Natures Own; Phoenix; Power; Quest; Reevecrest; Solgar; Vitalife)
	Bio C tablets (Blackmores)
	Biovit–C tablets (Bioceuticals)
	C Factors "1000" Plus tablets (Solgar)
	Cantassium Vitamin C Naturtabs (Larkhall)
	Earthlore Top C tablets (Lane)
	Ester–C tablets (Solgar)
	FSC Vitamin C tablets (Health & Diet)
	Gentle C tablets (Illingworth)
	Health Aid Super Vitamin C tablets (Pharmadass)
	Healthcrafts High Potency Vitamin C tablets (Ferrosan Healthcare)
	Redoxon Effervescent tablets (Roche)
	Schiff Vitamin C tablets (Weider)
	Super C tablets (Health Plus)
	Super Vitamin C tablets (Natural Flow)
1500 mg:	Vitamin C tablets (Lamberts; Natures Best; Solgar; Vitalife)
	Big C tablets (Illingworth)
	Cantassium Vitamin C Naturtabs (Larkhall)
	Health Aid Mega Vitamin C tablets (Pharmadass)

Mega C tablets (Natural Flow)

Vitamin D
400 units: Vitamin D Softgels (Solgar)
             FSC Vitamin D capsules (Health & Diet)
1000 units: Vitamin D Softgels (Solgar)

Vitamin E
10 units: Ephynal tablets (Roche)
50 units: Earthlore Vitamin E tablets (Lane)
75 units: Vita-E gels (Bioglan)
             Vita-E gelucaps (Bioglan)
100 units: Vitamin E capsules (Blackmores; Gerard; Healthilife; Lifeplan; Natures Aid; Natures Best; Natures Own; Power; Solgar)
             Vitamin E tablets (Blackmores)
             Cantassium Vitamin E capsules (Larkhall)
             Earthlore Fort-e-Vite capsules (Lane)
             Ephynal tablets (Roche)
             FSC Vitamin E capsules (Health & Diet)
             Healthcrafts Vitamin E capsules (Ferrosan Healthcare)
             Healthwise Vitamin E capsules (Illingworth)
150 units: Food State Vitamin E tablets (Natures Own)
200 units: Vitamin E capsules (Callanish; Gerard; Healthilife; Lamberts; Lifeplan; Natural Flow; Natures Aid; Natures Best; Natures Own; Phoenix; Power; Quest; Vitalia)
             Vitamin E Softgels (Solgar)
             Vitamin E Vegicaps (Solgar)
             Bio-E capsules (Bio-Health)
             Cantassium Vitamin E capsules (Larkhall)
             Cantassium Vitamin E Naturtabs (Larkhall)
             Capseco Vitamin E capsules (Brithealth)
             Earthlore Fort-e-Vite plus capsules (Lane)
             Ephynal tablets (Roche)
             Healthcrafts Vitamin E tablets (Ferrosan Healthcare)
             Healthwise Vitamin E capsules (Illingworth)
             Seven Seas Super Vitamin E capsules (Seven Seas)
             Vita-E gels (Bioglan)
             Vita-E succinate tablets (Bioglan)
250 units: Vitamin E capsules (Blackmores; Lamberts)
             Vitamin E tablets (Blackmores)
             FSC Vitamin E capsules (Health & Diet)
             Sanatogen Vitamin E capsules
400 units: Vitamin E capsules (Callanish; Lamberts; Lifeplan; Natural Flow; Natures Aid; Natures Best; Natures Own; Phoenix; Power; Quest; Solgar; Vitalia)
             Vitamin E Softgels (Solgar)
             Vitamin E tablets (Natural Flow)
             Health Aid Vitamin E capsules (Pharmadass)
             Schiff Vitamin E capsules (Weider)
             Vita-E gels (Bioglan)

500 units:	Vitamin E capsules (Blackmores; Healthilife; Natures Aid; Vitalife)
	Vitamin E tablets (Blackmores; Health Plus) Cantassium Vitamin E capsules (Larkhall)
	Earthlore Fort-e-Vite Super Plus capsules (Lane)
	Healthwise Vitamin E capsules (Illingworth)
525 units:	Bio-E Vitamin tablets (Pharma-Nord)
600 units:	Vitamin E capsules (Lamberts; Natures Best)
	Vitamin E tablets (Solgar)
	Brithealth Vitamin E capsules (Britannia)
	Cantassium Vitamin E capsules (Larkhall)
	FSC Vitamin E capsules (Health & Diet)
1000 units:	Vitamin E capsules (Healthilife; Lamberts; Lifeplan; Natural Flow; Natures Best; Phoenix; Power; Quest; Solgar; Vitalia)
	Vitamin E Softgels (Solgar)
	Biovit-E capsules (Bio-Health)
	Cantassium Vitamin E capsules (Larkhall)
	Earthlore Fort-e-Vite capsules (Lane)
	FSC Vitamin E capsules (Health & Diet)
	Healthcrafts Vitamin E tablets (Ferrosan Healthcare)
	Healthwise Vitamin E capsules (Illingworth)
	Vita-E succinate powder (Bioglan)
	Vital E capsules (Vitalife)

Vitamin K

100 µg:	Vitamin K tablets (Solgar)

Zinc

Note: Elemental zinc content per capsule or tablet is given in brackets where stated on product labels.
Available from:

Bioceuticals:	Super Zinc-C lozenges (50 mg)
	Zincosol Effervescent tablets (50 mg)
Bio-Health:	Pure-Fill Chelated Zinc capsules (4 mg)
	Pure-Fill Zinc Plus Formula capsules (15 mg)
Ferrosan Healthcare:	Healthcrafts Aminochel Zinc tablets (1.3 mg)
	Healthcrafts High Potency Aminochel Zinc tablets (5 mg)
	Healthcrafts Aminochel Zinc One-a-Day tablets (15 mg)
	Healthcrafts Zinc Gluconate tablets (4 mg)
Goldshield:	Z Span capsules (22.5 mg)
Health & Diet:	FSC Zinc tablets (4 mg)
	Zinc lozenges (3.5 mg)
	Zinc Picolinate capsules (30 mg)
Healthilife:	Amino Acid Chelated Zinc capsules (4 mg)
	Mega Zinc lozenges (11.2 mg)
Health Plus:	Ziman Plus tablets (20 mg)
Illingworth:	Healthwise Zinc Gluconate tablets (6.5 mg)
Lamberts:	Zinc Amino Acid Chelate tablets (15 mg)
	Chelated Zinc tablets (30 & 50 mg)

	Zinc Plus lozenges (7 mg)
	Zinc Citrate capsules (15 & 50 mg)
	DuoZinc liquid (15 mg/5 ml)
	Zinc Amino Acid Chelate capsules (50 mg)
Lane:	Zinc Supplement tablets (10 mg)
Larkhall:	Zinc with Mins Naturtabs (10 mg)
	B13 Zinc Naturtabs (100 mg)
	Zinc lozenges (25 mg)
	Zinc + B6 drops
Lifeplan:	Quadrazinc tablets (30 mg)
	Supazinc tablets (15 mg)
	Zinc Superactive tablets (10 mg)
Medo:	Zincomed capsules (50 mg)
Natural Flow:	Zinc Chewable lozenges (10 mg)
	Zinc tablets (10 & 50 mg)
Natures Aid:	Zinc Gluconate tablets (4 mg)
Natures Best:	Zincatest liquid
	Zinc Plus lozenges
	Zinc Plus Copper capsules
	Zinc Citrate capsules (15 mg)
	Chelated Zinc tablets (15 mg)
Natures Own:	Zinc Orotate tablets (2.4 mg; 6.4 mg; 16 mg)
	Food State tablets Zinc/Copper (15 mg/1 mg)
Pharmadass:	Health Aid Zinc Sulphate tablets (45 mg)
Phoenix:	Bio-Enhanced Zinc 20 tablets (20 mg)
	Zinc Citrate 50 tablets (50 mg)
Quest:	Synergistic Zinc tablets (20 mg)
Seven Seas:	Berries Zinc with Vitamin C capsules (1 mg)
Solgar:	Chelated Zinc tablets (22 mg)
	Flavo Zinc lozenges (23 mg)
	Zinc Citrate capsules (30 mg)
	Zinc "50" tablets (50 mg)
	Zinc Picolinate tablets (22 mg)
Vitalia:	Zinc Amino Acid Chelated tablets (15 mg)

Note: Supplements are also made by Asda, Boots, Lloyds, Numark, Sainsbury, Superdrug, Tesco and Unichem.

Multiple formulations

Antioxidants

Product Name and Manufacturer	Betacarotene (mg)	Vitamin C (mg)	Vitamin E (mg)	Selenium (µg)
Beta Pro (Natural Flow)	15	50	50	25
Beta-Max Carotene (Natures Best)	15	500	100	50
Betasec (Lamberts)	15	500	100	50
Body Protect (Jessup)	15	200	80	
Protector (Redoxon)	15	150	75	
Pulse (Seven Seas)	12	100	40	
Sanatogen (Roche)	6	200	100	
Selenium ACE (Wassen)[1]		90	45	100
Solgar Antioxidant	4.5	600	250	75

1. With vitamin A 450 µg

Vitamins A and D

Manufacturer	Vitamin A (units)	Vitamin D (units)
Lamberts	10 000	400
Natures Best	5000	400
Phoenix	10 000	400
Quest	7500	400
Seven Seas	2500	300
Solgar	7500	300

Vitamins A, C and D

Product Name and Manufacturer	Vitamin A (units)	Vitamin C (mg)	Vitamin D (units)
Haliborange (Reckitt & Colman)	2500	30	100
Healthcrafts SuperTed (Ferrosan Healthcare)	2500	30	100
Minadex tablets (Seven Seas)	1500	30	200

Vitamin B complex

Product Name and Manufacturer	B$_1$ (mg)	B$_2$ (mg)	Niacin (mg)	B$_6$ (mg)	B$_{12}$ (µg)	Fol (µg)	Pa (mg)	Biotin (µg)
Becosym (Roche)	5	2	20	2				
Becosym Forte (Roche)	15	15	50	10				
Benerva Compound (Roche)	1	1	15					
Berocca (Roche)[1]	11	14	47	8	9		22	130
Bio-Health								
Extra "B"	3	4	40	5	5	500	16	10
B Complex (High potency)	30	40	50	50	10	300	50	10
Evans B Complex	3.9	5	30	4.1	4	300	9.2	
Gerard								
Vitamin B Complex	25	20	20	25	5	100	20	20
Healthcrafts (Ferrosan Healthcare)								
Compleat Vitamin B/3tab	1.2	1.6	18	2	2	300	6	30
Super Compleat Vitamin B	4.8	6.4	72	9	5	300	65	3
PRN Mega-B Complex	100	100	100	100	5	300	90	100
Healthlife								
Vitamin B Complex	0.5	0.7	18	0.9	5	300	0.2	3
Super Vitamin B Complex	10	10	50	10	10	300	10	
Healthwise Vitamin B								
Complex (Illingworth)	10	10	30	6	10	200	9.2	
Health Aid (Pharmadass)								
Full Vitamin B	50	50	50	50	10	50	50	50
B Complex Supreme	10	10	10	10	10	100	10	10
Strong B50	50	50	50	50	10	50	50	50
Mega B99	99	99	99	99	19	99	99	99
Health Plus								
B Complex	50	50	50	50	10	100	50	100
Lamberts								
Vitamin B-50 Complex								
Tables	50	50	50	50	50	100	50	50
Capsules	50	50	50	50	50	400	50	50

Vitamin B complex cont.

Product Name and Manufacturer	B_1 (mg)	B_2 (mg)	Niacin (mg)	B_6 (mg)	B_{12} (µg)	Fol (µg)	Pa (mg)	Biotin (µg)
Vitamin B-100 Complex	100	100	100	100	100	100	100	100
Natural Flow								
B Complex	10	10	50	10	10	100	15	20
Mega B Complex	75	75	75	75	10	100	75	75
Natures Best								
Vital B-Complex	10	10	60	10	10	400	80	100
B-50 Complex	50	50	50	50	50	100	50	50
B-100 Complex	100	100	100	100	100	100		
Natures Own								
Vitamin B Complex Plus	50	25	50	50	5	100	50	50
Phoenix								
Mega B-50 Complex								
Tablets	50	50	50	50	50	400	50	50
Capsules	50	50	50	50	50	1000	50	50
Mega B-100	100	100	100	100	100	400	100	100
Quest								
Multi B Complex[2]	8	10	50	8	15	400	30	10
Super Mega B+C[1]	39	50	50	41	50	400	50	50
Mega B50	39	50	50	41	50	400	50	50
Mega B100	79	100	100	82	100	400	100	100
Sanatogen (Roche)								
Vitamin B Complex	1.2	1.6	18	2	2	300		
Seven Seas								
Vitamin B Complex	15	10	20	40	10	100	10	6
Solgar								
B Complex with C[1]	10	10	100	10	25	100	100	25
Formula B-Complex "50"	50	50	50	50	50	400	50	50
Formula B-Complex "100"	100	100	100	100	100	400	100	100

1. With vitamin C 1000mg
2. With vitamin C 500mg
Abbreviations: Fol = Folic Acid; Pa = Pantothenic Acid

Multivitamins

Columns are grouped under **Vitamin** (A … Bio) and **Mineral** (Fe … Chr).

Product	A μg	C mg	D μg	E mg	K μg	B_1 mg	B_2 mg	Nia mg	B_6 mg	B_{12} μg	Fol μg	Pa mg	Bio μg	Fe mg	Zn mg	Ca mg	Mg mg	K mg	P mg	Cu mg	Se μg	I μg	Mn mg	Mo μg	Chr μg
Abidec drops, 0.6 ml (Warner-Lambert)	1200	50	10			1	0.4	5	0.5																
Adexolin drops																									
0.14 ml (Seven Seas)	225	15	5																						
Allbee with C (Robins)		300				15	10	50	5	5		10													
BC 500 (Whitehall)		500				25	12.5	100	10	5		20													
Bio-caps (Bio-Health)	250	80	2.5	30		2.5	3	30	2.5			12	5	12	2	50	10			1.0		140			
Berocca (Roche)		1000				11	14	46	8	9	300	22	130			120									
Biovital (Roche)																									
Tablets		20				0.6	0.6	10	1	2				32.5									0.15		
Liquid 20 ml		20				0.6	2.6	10	1	2				12									0.6		
Boots																									
Multivitamins	750	30	2.5	5		1.2	1.6	18	1	2		4.6													
Multivitamins with iron	750	30	2.5	5		1.2	1.6	18	1	2		4.6		12	4					0.75		140	1		
Multivitamins, minerals and ginseng	750	30	2.5	2.5		1.2	1.6	18	0.5	2		2.3		12	0.75	10	2.5	1		0.375		140	0.5	100	
Multivitamins for children	750	30	2.5	7		1.2	1.6	18	0.75	2		3.7													
Multivitamin																									
Syrup, 10 ml	240	16	3.25	4		0.75	0.94	4	0.5	2		2.67													
Chewable	750	30	2.5	7		1.2	1.6	18	0.75																
Chewable A, C & D	750	30	2.5																						
Concavit (Wallace)																									
Capsules	1500	40	10	2		2.5	2.5	20	1	2		5													
Drops, ml	3000	100	20			4	2	25	2			4													
Liquid, 5 ml	1500	50	10			2	1	12.5	1			2													
Davitet Drops (Eastern)																									
Liquid, 0.6 ml	1500	50	10	5		1	0.4	5	0.5			1	4												
Dynavites (Healthilife)	750	75	5			1.5	2	15	1.5	2				14	1		1.3					150	0.3		
Evans																									
Multivitamins plus Iron	750	30	6.25	5		1.3	1.7	19	0.8	4	10	4.6		12											
Femia-9 (Seven Seas)		60		30					60	2	300			12	4							140			
Feroglobin B12 (Vitabiotics)									5	10	500			24	12					2					
Forceval (Unigreg)																									
Capsules	750	60	10	5		1.2	1.6	18	2	3	300	4	100	12	15	100	30	4	77	2	50	140	3	250	200
Junior capsules	495	25	2.5	5		1	1	3.3	0.3	2	100	2	50	5	5		1			1	25	75	1.25	50	50

Multivitamins cont.

Product	Vitamin													Mineral											
	A µg	C mg	D µg	E mg	K µg	B1 mg	B2 mg	Nia mg	B6 mg	B12 µg	Fol µg	Pa mg	Bio µg	Fe mg	Zn mg	Ca mg	Mg mg	K mg	P mg	Cu mg	Se µg	I µg	Mn mg	Mo µg	Chr µg
Genesis (Wassen)	450	30	2.5	10		5	5		50					12	8		145	8		0.5	25	140	2		25
Gericaps (Pharmadass)	1500	50	10	10		5.0	5.0	15	0.5	1		5		10	0.5	145	1	5	110	1		100			
Gerimax (Vitalia)	900	45	10	12		1.5	1.8	20	2	3	100	10		18	15					2	125	150	3.8	250	125
Gevral (Lederle)	1500	50	12.5	10		5.0	15	0.5	1			5		10	0.5	145	1	5	110	1		100	1		
Gynovite Plus (Lamberts)	250	30	2	66.7	5.0	1.7	1.7	3.3	3.3	21	66.7	1.7	21	3	2.5	83.3	100			0.3	33.3	25	1.7		33.3
Hallborange (Reckitt & Colman)																									
With vitamins A, C and D	750	30	2.5																						
Multivitamins with iron & calcium	750	60	2.5	6		1.2	1.5	10	1	2	300	5		6		135									
Health Aid (Pharmadass)																									
Multivitamins and minerals	750	50	10	12		1.8	2.4	18	3	3	300	2.3		18	15		2								
Healthcrafts (Ferrosan Healthcare)																									
Multivitamins with iron and calcium	750	30	2.5	10		1.2	1.6	18	2	2	300														
Mega-Multis	750	300	6.2	150		48	64	72	60	5	300	60		12			4	50	12	0.33			140	100	0.7
Chewable multi-vitamins/2	750	120	2.5	30		3.6	4.8	36	4	2	300	10	100												
Super Gev-E	750	90	6.25	80		6.0	4.0		1	2	300	10	1	15	2	65	1	1	50	0.4	140	140	0.01		100
Healthwise																									
Multivitamin & Mineral Ultimate	600	60	5	25		5	5	25	7.5	35	200	10	2	3	0.4	60	0.4		27	0.1	150	150	0.5	100	
Multivitamins Plus	300	250	10	100		100	100	100	100		400	100	100		1.5	10	1.4			0.01	150	150	0.6		0.5
Iron Jelloids (Smith-Kline Beecham)		4.2				0.2	0.3	1.7						20											
Ladytone (Vitabiotics)	750	30		15		12	3	20	8	6	200	6	150	21.5	1.5		20			0.5		75	1		
Lamberts																									
Multiple Vitamins & Minerals	2500	200	10	5		10	10	100	5	5	200	5		15	1.5	105	6	5			75		1		

Multivitamins cont.

Product	A μg	C mg	D μg	E mg	K μg	B_1 mg	B_2 mg	Nia mg	B_6 mg	B_{12} μg	Fol μg	Pa mg	Bio μg	Fe mg	Zn mg	Ca mg	Mg mg	K mg	P mg	Cu mg	Se μg	I μg	Mn mg	Mo μg	Chr μg
Larkhall																									
Cantamega 1000	750	100	6.25	50	10	10	10	25	15	5	25	25	20	2	1.2	141	6.6	2		0.3	5	130	0.4	100	20
Cantamega 2000	2250	300	10	200	10	79	100	100	82	100	400	100	100	2.6	2.4	80.7	39.8	2		0.3	10	224	1	100	40
Foresight Minerals														5	6.5	31	15	1.25					4		1200
Foresight Vitamins	333	100	2.5	50	250	4	5.5	25	12.5	10	200		17.5												
Trufree Vits & Mins	415	100	5	70	100	3.9	5	50	12.3	10	100	50	100	1.3	1.5	35	7.6			0.03		50	1.5	100	200
Lifeplan																									
Formula 8 Multi-vitamins without iron	750	30	5	5		1.2	1.6	18		2	300														
Formula 8 Multi-vitamins + iron	750	30	2.5	5		1.2	1.6	18		2	300			12								140			
Lloyds																									
Multivitamins	750	50	6.25	4		1.2	1.8	12														100			
Multivitamins with iron	750	50	6.25	4			1.8	12						20								100			
Multivitamins with minerals	750	30	2.5	25			1.6	18		2	300	5	0.5	12	3.5	30	0.5	0.5	23	0.2		100	0.05	50	
Maxvit Lanes	600	50	5.0	25		2.0	3.0	25	4	2	200	5	1	10	10	60			27	0.5					
Menopace (Vitabiotics)	750	45	5.0	30		20	5.0	20	40	9	400	30	30	12	15	100	100			1	100	225	2		50
Minadex (Seven Seas) Children's vitamins	500	30	5.0	5.0			2	18																	
Multivitamin syrup for children, 10 ml	1200	35	10	3		1.4	1.7	18	0.7		300														
Multiron (Vitabiotics)	750	30	5	5		10	2	20	2	10	300	3		18	8		10	5		0.5	100	140	0.5		50
Multiplex (Gerard)	750	60	5	40		10	10	25	10	4	100	5	10		1	6	0.07	1		0.5	12	75	1		15
Natural Flow Mega Multi	2500	250	10	200		75	75	75	75	10	200	75	75	10	15	50	8	10				150	6		
Natures Aid																									
Multivitamin + Mineral	750	75	5	5		1.5	2	18	1.5	2	300	1	4	12	1	40	1.25	2				140	0.5		
Natures Best																									
Multi-Guard	1775	150	10	100		25	25	100	25	100	400	50	150	10	15	25	7			2	200	150	5	500	200
Megavit/75	2250	250	10	150		75	75	75	75	75	400	75	75	1	1.5	10	1.5	1		0.02	25	150	0.6		
Natures Own																									
Multivitamin	750	50	5	100		20	20	30	30	5	100	20	50												

Multivitamins cont.

Product	Vitamin													Mineral											
	A µg	C mg	D µg	E mg	K µg	B$_1$ mg	B$_2$ mg	Nia mg	B$_6$ mg	B$_{12}$ µg	Fol µg	Pa mg	Bio µg	Fe mg	Zn mg	Ca mg	Mg mg	K mg	P mg	Cu mg	Se µg	I µg	Mn mg	Mo µg	Chr µg
Numark																									
Multivitamins	750	30	2.5	2		2	2	20	2	2	300														
Multivitamins with iron	750	30	2.5	2		2	2	20	2	2	300			12											
Multivitamins with extra Vitamin C	750	200	2.5	2		2	2	20	2	2	300														
Octovit (Goldshield)	750	30	2.5	10		1	1.5	20	2	2	300			10	5	10									
Omega H3 (Vitabiotics)	1667	60	5	20		20	5	25	10	9	500	10	30	15		26					100	150		50	50
Optivite (Lamberts)	375	250	0.4	16.6		3.4	4.2	4.25		10.4	33.3	4.2	10.4	2.5	4.2	21	41.6	7.9		0.08	16.6	12.5			16.6
Orovite (SmithKline Beecham)		100				50	5	200	5																
Orovite 7 (SmithKline Beecham)	750	60	2.5			1.4	1.7	18	2	9	500														
Perfectil (Vitabiotics)	750	30	25	30		10	5	18	20		500	50	45	18	15		50			2	100	200	2		50
Pharmaton (Windsor Healthcare)	1200	60	10	10		2.0	2.0	15	1	1		10		10	1	90	10	8	70	1			1		
Phillips (Phillips Yeast)																									
Iron Tonic						0.16	0.3	2						20											
Tonic Yeast		10				0.1	0.2	1.4	0.09			0.01													
Phyllosan (SmithKline Beecham)	750	5	2.5			0.16	0.3	8.5						15	10	125	20					100			
Pregnacare (Vitabiotics)	750	30	2.5	20		3		20	6	6	400			24	15		120	10	63	1	25	150			25
Premence (Vitabiotics)	750	60	30	30	200	12	2	36	45	5	300	50		15	10		60			1		100			
Red Kooga Ginseng with multivitamins and minerals	750	30	2.5	5		1.2	1.6	18	2	2	300	5		18	15	140		100		0.5	50	140	1		
Quest	750	150	10	50		39	50	50	41	50	200	50	50												
Sanatogen (Roche)																									
Multivitamins	750	30	2.5	5		1.2	1.6	18	2	2	300														
Multivitamins with iron	750	30	2.5	5		1.2	1.6	18	2	2	300			12											
Multivitamins with calcium	750	30	2.5			1.2	1.6	18	2	2	300					92									
Multivitamins with evening primrose oil	600	30	2.5	10		1.2	1.6	18	2	2	300	6	150												
Children's	750	30	2.5																						
Children's vitamins and minerals	240	20	2.5											3		85						110			

Multivitamins cont.

Product	\$A\$ µg	\$C\$ mg	\$D\$ µg	\$E\$ mg	\$K\$ µg	\$B_1\$ mg	\$B_2\$ mg	Nia mg	\$B_6\$ mg	\$B_{12}\$ µg	Fol µg	Pa mg	Bio µg	Fe mg	Zn mg	Ca mg	Mg mg	\$K\$ mg	\$P\$ mg	Cu mg	Se µg	\$I\$ µg	Mn mg	Mo µg	Chr µg
Sanatogen (Roche) cont.																									
Teen	400	22	2.5	5		0.6	0.9	10	10	1	150			11.4		120	50								
Vegetarian			5				1.6		2	4	300			12	7	120				0.6					
Selenium ACE (Wassen International)	450	90		45																	100				
Seven Seas																									
Multivitamins and minerals	750	40	2.5	30		2.3	2.0	20	8	2	12.55		0.5	12	4	20	0.5	0.5	15	0.2		140	0.005	50	
Multivitamin berries with evening primrose oil	750	30	6.25	10		1.1	1.7	12	1																
Multivitamins from natural sources	750	20	2.5	5																					
Multivitamins from natural sources with iron	750	20	2.5	5										12											
Solgar																									
Daily Gold Pack	3300	600	10	400		100	100	100	100	100	400	100	400	10	10	500	250	99	200	0.2	50	150	10	60	20
Formula VM-75	2500	250	10	150		75	75	75	75	75	400	75	75	1	1.5	9	1.3	18			10	150	0.6		
Super Plenamins (3M Healthcare)	1500	40	7.5	1.5		2.25	2.25	20	0.85	2		0.5		18	1	75	15	3	58	0.75		150	1.25		
Supradyn, 2 capsules (Roche)	1500	150	10	10		15	5	50	10	5	300	11.6	250	15	with Ca, Fe, Mg, P, Cu, Zn, Mo, Mn										
Totavit (Cupal)	1200	30	10	1		1.5	1.2	10	0.5							24		18.5		0.1					
Unichem																									
Multivitamins	750	30	2.5	4		1.2	1.6	18	2													140			
Multivitamins & Iron	750	30	2.5	4		1.2	1.6	18	2					12	3.5	100			50			140			
Multivitamins & Minerals	750	30	2.5	25		1.2	1.6	18	7.5	2	300	5	0.5	12	30	100	0.5	0.5	80	0.2		140	0.05	50	
Vitalia																									
Multivitamins and minerals	1000	60	5	10		1.5	1.7	19	2.2	3	100	6			15					2.5	125	150			125
Multivitamins and minerals with iron	1000	60	5	10		1.5	1.7	19	2.2	3	100	6		18	15					2.5	125	150			125

Column groups: columns \$A\$–Bio fall under **Vitamin**; columns Fe–Chr fall under **Mineral**.

Multivitamins cont.

Product	Vitamin													Mineral											
	A µg	C mg	D µg	E mg	K µg	B$_1$ mg	B$_2$ mg	Nia mg	B$_6$ mg	B$_{12}$ µg	Fol µg	Pa mg	Bio µg	Fe mg	Zn mg	Ca mg	Mg mg	K mg	P mg	Cu mg	Se µg	I µg	Mn mg	Mo µg	Chr µg
Vitamins Capsules BPC	750	15	7.5			1	0.5	7.5																	
The VV Pack (Health Plus)	2500	1250	10	100		75	75	75	75	10	100	75	100	13.8	10.7								6.2		20
Vykmin (SmithKline Beecham)	750	30	10			1.2	1.6	18		2	300														
Yeast-Vite (SmithKline Beecham)						0.17	0.17	1.75																	

Abbreviations: Bio = biotin; Fol = Folic acid; Nia = niacin; Pa = pantothenic acid.

Note: All figures are for a unit dose except where stated, eg Abidec, 0.6 ml; Supradyn, 2 capsules.

Chapter 58
Appendix 2: Medically recognized indications for vitamins and minerals

Vitamins and minerals are authoritatively recommended either as a means of preventing disease or to exert a pharmacological effect. The use of folic acid pre-conceptually and in early pregnancy to prevent neural tube defects is one example of an accepted prophylactic approach. (The use of folic acid for this purpose is covered in more detail in the main text (Chapter 21) as many women now buy folic acid over the counter.)

Vitamins and minerals may be prescribed on the NHS to prevent or treat deficiency and in conditions which may lead to deficiency states. These include:

- severe malabsorption (coeliac disease, regional enteritis, tropical sprue),
- severe prolonged intestinal infection and/or persistent diarrhoea,
- gastrectomy,
- pancreatic disease,
- hepatic/biliary tract disease,
- prolonged fever and/or infection,
- burns, severe wounds and major surgery,
- cancer,
- AIDS,
- renal disease,
- chronic haemodialysis, and
- total parenteral nutrition (TPN)

There are also a number of specific clinical disorders in which the use of higher doses of specific vitamins and minerals may be indicated. Further specific information is given in the Tables in the following pages.

Table 58.1 Some clinical indications for specific vitamins and minerals

Substance	Indications
Vitamins	
Vitamins A, D, E and K	Clearly diagnosed fat malabsorption syndromes
Vitamin B group	Alcoholism
Thiamine	Maple syrup urine disease; pyruvate carboxylase deficiency; hyperalaninaemia
Riboflavin	Inborn error of flavin metabolism
Niacin	Hartnup disease
Nicotinic acid	Hyperlipidaemia
Folic acid	Prophylaxis in pregnancy; folate-deficient megaloblastic anaemia; congenital megaloblastic anaemia; homocysteinuria; formiminotransferase deficiency
Biotin	Biotinidase deficiency
Vitamin B$_6$	Pyridoxine dependency syndrome; idiopathic sideroblastic anaemia; congenital metabolic dysfunction (cystanthionuria; hyperoxaluria; homocysteinuria; xanthurenic aciduria); isoniazid neuropathy
Vitamin B$_{12}$	Pernicious anaemia; transcobalamin II deficiency; methlymalonic aciduria; homocysteinuria; hypomethioninaemia; subacute degeneration of the spinal cord
Vitamin D	See Table 58.2
Vitamin E	Familial isolated vitamin E deficiency; premature or low birth weight infants (controversial)
Vitamin K	Prophylaxis against vitamin K deficiency bleeding in infants (see Table 58.3)
Minerals	
Calcium	Hyperphosphataemia; hypocalcaemic tetany; hypoparathyroidism;
Copper	Menke's disease
Magnesium	Hyperaldosteronism; hyperparathyroidectomy; post-parathyroidectomy; serious arrhythmias (controversial); myocardial infarction (controversial)
Potassium	Secondary hyperaldosteronism
Zinc	Acrodermatitis enteropathica
Miscellaneous	
Betacarotene	Erythropoietic protoporphyria
Carnitine	Genetic carnitine deficiency; liver/renal failure; organic aciduria
Fish oil (Maxepa)	Severe hypertriglyceridaemia
Gamma-linolenic acid	Atopic eczema (Epogam); Mastalgia (Efamast)

Note: With the exception of folic acid (for prophylaxis in pregnancy), supplements should not be sold over the counter for these indications (medical supervision is essential).

Table 58.2 Recognized Indications[1] for Vitamin D Substances

Clinical indications	Ergocalciferol (Calciferol; Vitamin D2)	Alfacalcidol (1a-hydroxy cholecalciferol)	Calcitriol (1, 25, dihydroxy cholecalciferol)	Dihydro-tachysterol
Prevention of Vitamin D deficiency	●			
Treatment of Vitamin D deficiency	●			
Vitamin D malabsorption	●	●		
Vitamin D dependent rickets	●	●		
Vitamin D resistant rickets	●	●		
Hypoparathyroidism	●	●		●
Renal osteodystrophy		●	●	
Neonatal hypocalcaemia		●		
Hypocalcaemic tetany				●

1. Based on UK Product Licences
Note: Vitamin D requires hydroxylation in the kidney to its active form. Therefore the hydroxylated derivatives, alfacalcidol or calcitriol should be prescribed if patients with severe renal impairment require vitamin D.

Table 58.3 Recommended[1] doses of oral[2] vitamin K in infants for the prevention of haemorrhagic disease

	Dose
On the day of birth (all infants)	500 µg of Konakion[3] as a single dose or two 250 µg doses
	then:
Breast fed infants	200 µg Konakion weekly for 26 weeks, or 500 µg Konakion at the 7–10 day check and the 4–6 week check, or 50 µg daily for the first 26 weeks
Bottle fed infants	None (after initial dose), because infant formulas have added vitamin K

1. Recommendations of the British Paediatric Association (1992).
2. If the oral route is not available or thought to be unreliable vitamin K is given by injection (Konakion 100 µg) and further doses given orally to breast fed infants or by injection if the oral route remains unavailable.
3. Konakion is a formulation containing vitamin K.

Chapter 59
Appendix 3: Directory of manufacturers

Abbott Laboratories Ltd, Abbott House, Norden Rd, Maidenhead, Berkshire SL6 4XE. Tel: 01628 773355. *Fax: 01795 580404*

ASTA Medica Ltd, 168 Cowley Rd, Cambridge CB4 4DL. Tel: 01223 423434. *Fax: 01223 420943*

Astra Pharmaceuticals Ltd, Home Park Estate, Kings Langley, Hertfordshire WD4 8DH. Tel: 01923 266191. *Fax: 01923 260341*

Biocare Ltd, 54 Northfield Rd, Kings Norton, Birmingham B30 1JH. Tel: 0121 433 3727

Bioceuticals Ltd, 26 Zennor Rd, London SW12 OPS. Tel: 0181-675 5664. *Fax: 0181-675 2257*

Bioglan Laboratories Ltd, 1 The Cam Centre, Wilbury Way, Hitchin, Hertfordshire SG4 OTW. Tel: 01462 438444. *Fax: 01462 421242*

Bio-Health Ltd, Culpeper Close, Medway City Estate, Rochester, Kent ME2 4HU. Tel: 01634 290115. *Fax: 0634 290761*

Blackmores Laboratories Ltd, Unit 7, Poyle Tech Centre, Willow Rd, Poyle, Colnbrook, Buckinghamshire SL3 0PD. Tel: 01753 683185. *Fax: 01753 684663*

Brithealth Ltd, Weltech Centre, Ridgeway, Welwyn Garden City, Hertfordshire AL7 2AA. Tel: 01707 328118. *Fax: 01707 372964*

Callanish Ltd, Breasclete, Isle of Lewis PA86 9ED. Tel: 01851 621366

Cedar Health Ltd, Pepper Rd, Hazel Grove, Stockport, Cheshire SK7 5BW. Tel: 0161 483 1235. *Fax: 0161 456 4321*

Chemist Brokers (division of Food Brokers Ltd), Food Broker House, Northarbour Rd, North Harbour, Portsmouth, Hampshire PO6 3TD. Tel: 01705 219900. *Fax: 01705 219222*

CIBA Laboratories, Wimblehurst Rd, Horsham, West Sussex RH12 4AB. Tel: 01403 272827. *Fax: 01403 323054*

Colgate-Palmolive Ltd, Guildford Business Park, Middleton Rd, Guildford, Surrey GU2 5LZ. Tel: 01483 302222. *Fax: 01483 303003*

Consolidated Chemicals Ltd, Abbey Rd, The Industrial Estate, Wrexham, Clwyd LL13 9PW. Tel: 01978 661351. *Fax: 01978 661673*

Dental Health Products Ltd, Broughton House, 33 Earl St, Maidstone, Kent, ME14 1PF. Tel 01622 762269. *Fax: 01622 764046*

Efamol Ltd, Units 26–29, Surrey Technology Centre, The Research Park, Guildford, Surrey GU2 5YH. Tel: 01483 304441. *Fax: 01483 304437*.

Emperor Ginseng Co Ltd, 2 Water Run Farm Cottage, Gipping Back Rd, Stow Upland, Stowmarket, Suffolk IP14 4BA. Tel: 01449 676175.

English Grains Healthcare, Swains Park Industrial Estate, Park Rd, Overseal, Swadlincote, Derbyshire DE12 6JT. Tel: 01283 221616. *Fax: 01283 550185*

Evans Medical Ltd, Evans House, Regent Park, Kingston Rd, Leatherhead, Surrey, KT22 7PQ. Tel: 01372 364000. *Fax: 01372 364050*

Evening Primrose Oil Co Ltd, 116–120 London Rd, Headington, Oxford OX3 9BBA. Tel: 01865 750717. *Fax: 01865 68826*

Ferrosan Healthcare Ltd, Beaver House, York House, Byfleet, Surrey KT14 7HN. Tel: 01932 336366. *Fax: 01932 336023*

Food Supplement Co Ltd: (see Health & Diet Food Co Ltd)

Galen Ltd, Seagoe Industrial Estate, Craigavon, Northern Ireland BT63 5UA. Tel: 01762 334974. *Fax: 01762 350206*

Gerard House Ltd, 475 Capability Green, Luton, Bedfordshire LU1 3LU Tel: 01582 487331. *Fax: 01582 484941*

Goldshield Pharmaceuticals Ltd, Bensham House, 324 Bensham Lane, Thornton Heath, Surrey CR7 7EQ. Tel: 0181-684 3664. *Fax: 0181-665 6433*

Health & Diet Food Co Ltd, Europa Trading Estate, Stoneclough Rd, Radcliffe, Manchester M26 9HE. Tel: 01204 707420. *Fax: 01204 73291*

Healthilife Ltd, Charlestown House, Baildon, Shipley, West Yorkshire BD17 7JS. Tel: 01274 595021. *Fax: 01274 581515*

Health Dynamics Ltd, Bolton Enterprise Centre, Washington St, Bolton, Lancashire BL3 5EA. Tel: 01204 24262. *Fax: 01204 35995*

Health Plus, PO Box 86, Seaford, East Sussex BN25 4ZW. Tel: 01323 492096. *Fax: 01323 490452*

Health World Ltd, 7 Falcon Court, St Martins Way, London SW17 0JH. Tel: 0181-944 0040. *Fax: 0181-944 0032*

Ideal Health plc, Paradise, Hemel Hempstead, Hertfordshire HP2 4TF. Tel: 01442 231155. *Fax: 01442 218180*

Illingworth Health Foods Ltd, York House, York St, Bradford, West Yorkshire BD8 0HR. Tel: 0274 488511. *Fax: 0274 541121*

Jessup Ltd, 27 Old Gloucester St, London WC1N 3XX

Lamberts Healthcare Ltd, 1 Lamberts Rd, Tunbridge Wells, Kent TN2 3EQ. Tel: 01892 564488. *Fax: 01892 515863*

Lane Health, GR, Products Ltd, Sisson Rd, Gloucester GL1 3QB. Tel: 0452 524012. *Fax: 01452 300105*

Larkhall Laboratories, 225 Putney Bridge Road, London SW15 2PY. Tel: 0181-874 1130. *Fax: 0181-871 0066*

Lederle Laboratories, Cyanamid House, Fareham Rd, Gosport, Hampshire PO13 0AS. Tel: 01329 224000. *Fax: 01329 220213*

Lewis Laboratories, PO Box 1804, Buckingham MK18 2LG. Tel: 01296 712151. *Fax: 01296 715643*

Lichtwer Pharma UK, Dominions House, Eton Pl, 64 High St, Burnham, Buckinghamshire SL1 7JT. Tel: 01628 605275. *Fax: 01628 605277*

Lifeplan Products, Elizabethan Way, Lutterworth, Leicestershire LE17 4ND. Tel: 014555 56281. *Fax: 01455 556261*

Life Stream Research (UK), Ash House, Stedham, Midhurst, West Sussex GU29 0PT. Tel: 01730 813642. *Fax: 01730 815109*

Link Pharmaceuticals Ltd, 41 Swan Walk, Horsham, West Sussex RH12 1HQ. Tel: 01403 272451. *Fax: 01403 218355*

Lusty's Natural Products Ltd (see Lane, GR, Health Products Ltd)

Man Shuen Hong (London), 80 Roll Gardens, Gants Hill, Essex IG2 6TL. Tel: 0181-550 9900. *Fax: 0181-551 8100*

Medo Pharmaceuticals Ltd, Schwarz House, East St, Chesham, Buckinghamshire HP5 1DG. Tel: 01494 772071. *Fax: 01494 773394*

Myplan Ltd, Manor House, 12a Castle St, Berkhamsted, Hertfordshire HP4 2BQ. Tel: 01442 862553

Napp Laboratories Ltd, Cambridge Science Park, Milton Rd, Cambridge, CB4 4GW. Tel: 01223 424444. *Fax: 01223 424441*

Natural Care, PO Box 100, Thornton Heath, Surrey CR7 7YP. Tel: 0181-665 9670. *Fax: 0181-689 3969*

Natural Flow Ltd, Green Farm, Burwash, East Sussex TN19 7LX. Tel. 01435 882482. *Fax: 01435 882929*

Natures Aid Health Products, Whitworth St, Wesham, Kirkham, Preston, Lancashire PR4 3AU. Tel: 01772 686231. *Fax: 01772 671688*

Natures Best, PO Box 1, 1 Lamberts Rd, Tunbridge Wells, Kent TN2 3EQ. Tel: 01892 34143. *Fax: 01892 515863*

Natures Own Ltd, 203–205 West Malvern Rd, West Malvern, Worcestershire WR14 4BB. Tel: 01684 892555. *Fax: 01684 892643*

Neutraceuticals (division of Three Spires Pharmaceuticals), The Orchard, Fenny Bentley, Derbyshire DE6 1LB. Tel 01335 29594

Novex Pharma Ltd, Innovex House, Reading Rd, Henley-on-Thames, Oxfordshire RG9 1EL. Tel: 01491 578171. *Fax: 01491 575057*

Oral-B Laboratories Ltd, Gatehouse Rd, Aylesbury, Bucks HP19 3ED. Tel 01296 432601. *Fax: 01296 434283*

Paines & Byrne Ltd, Brocades House, Pyrford House, West Byfleet, Surrey KT14 6RA. Tel: 01932 355405. *Fax: 01932 353458*

Parkwood Health Ltd, PO Box 1, 1 Lamberts Rd, Tunbridge Wells, Kent TN2 3EQ. Tel 0892 510559

Pharma-Nord (UK) Ltd, Spital Hall, Mitford, Morpeth NE61 3PI. Tel: 01670 519989. *Fax: 01670 513222*

Pharmadass Ltd, 16 Aintree Rd, Greenford Rd, Greenford, Middlesex UB6 7LA. Tel: 0181-991 0035. *Fax: 0181-997 3490*

Phillips Yeast Products Ltd, Park Royal Rd, London NW10 7JX. Tel: 0181-965 7533. *Fax: 0181-961 2610*

Phoenix Nutrition Ltd, Thorpe Close, Banbury, Oxon OX16 8SW. Tel: 01295 271311. *Fax: 01295 271818*

Power Health Products, 10 Central Ave, Airfield Estate, Pocklington, York Y04 2NR. Tel: 01759 302595. *Fax: 01759 304286*

Procter & Gamble Pharmaceuticals UK Ltd, Lovett House, Lovett Rd, Staines, Middlesex TW18 3AZ. Tel: 01784 495000. *Fax: 01784 495297*

Quest Vitamins Ltd, Unit 1, Premier Trading Estate, Dartmouth Middleway, Birmingham B7 4AT. Tel: 0121-359 0056. *Fax: 0121-359 0313*

Rainbow Light Nutritional Systems, 62 Wilson St, London EC2A 2BU

Reckitt & Colman Products, Dansom Lane, Hull, Humberside HU8 7DS. Tel: 01482 26151. *Fax: 01482 25322*

Reevecrest Health Care, 10 Central Avenue, Airfield Estate, Pocklington, North Yorkshire YO4 2NR. Tel: 01759 302595. *Fax: 01759 304286*

Regina Royal Jelly Ltd, 2a Alexandra Grove, Finchley, London N12 8NU. Tel: 0181-446 6644. *Fax: 0181-445 4551*

Rio Trading Company (Health) Ltd, 2 Centenary Estate, Hughes Road, Brighton East Sussex BN2 4AW. Tel: 01273 570987. *Fax: 01273 691226*

Roche Nicholas Consumer Healthcare, PO Box 8, Welwyn Garden City, Hertfordshire AL7 3AY. Tel: 01707 366000. *Fax: 01707 338297*

RP Drugs Ltd, RPD House, Yorkdale Industrial Park, Braithwaite St, Leeds, West Yorkshire LS11 9XE. Tel: 0113-244 1400. *Fax: 0113-246 0738*

Rybar Laboratories Ltd, Fosse House, East Anton Court, Icknield Way, Andover, Hampshire SP10 SRG. Tel: 01264 333455 *Fax: 01264 333460*

Sandoz Pharmaceuticals, Frimley Business Park, Frimley, Camberley, Surrey GU16 5SG. Tel: 0276 692255. *Fax: 0276 692508*

Sanofi Winthrop Ltd, 1 Onslow St, Guildford, Surrey GU1 4YS. Tel: 01483 505515. *Fax: 01483 35432*

Seton Healthcare Group plc, Turbiton House, Medlock St, Oldham, Lancashire OL1 3HS. Tel: 0161 652 2222. *Fax: 0161-626 9090*

Seven Seas Health Care Ltd, Hedon Rd, Marfleet, Kingston-upon-Hull, Humberside HU9 5NJ. Tel: 01482 75234. *Fax: 01482 74345*

Shire Pharmaceuticals Ltd, 1 Viscount Court, South Way, Andover, Hampshire SP10 5NW. Tel: 01264 333455. *Fax: 01264 333460*

Sinclair Pharmaceuticals Ltd, Borough Rd, Godalming, Surrey GU7 2AB. Tel: 01483 426644.

SmithKline Beecham Consumer Brands, St George's Ave, Weybridge, Surrey KT13 0DE. Tel: 01932 822000

Solgar Vitamins Ltd, Solgar House, Chiltern Commerce Centre, Asheridge Rd Industrial Park, Chesham, Buckinghamshire, England. Tel: 01494 791691. *Fax: 01494 792729*

Stafford-Miller Ltd, Broadwater Rd, Welwyn Garden City, Hertfordshire, AL7 3SP. Tel 01707 331001. *Fax: 01707 373370*

3M Healthcare Ltd, 3M House, 1 Morley Street, Loughborough, Leicestershire LE11 1EP. Tel: 01509 611611. *Fax: 01509 237288*

Tillomed Laboratories Ltd, Unit 2, Campus 5, Letchworth Business Park, Letchworth Garden City, Hertfordshire SG6 2JF. Tel: 01462 480344.

Unichem, Unichem House, Cox Lane, Chessington, Surrey KT9 1SN. Tel: 0181-391 2323. *Fax: 0181-974 1707*

Unigreg Ltd, Enterprise House, 181–185 Garth Rd, Morden, Surrey SM4 4LL. Tel 0181-330 1421. *Fax: 0181-330 6812*

Upjohn Ltd, Fleming Way, Crawley, West Sussex RH10 2LZ. Tel: 01293 531133. *Fax: 01293 536894*

Vitabiotics Ltd, Vitabiotics House, 3 Bashley Rd, London NW10 6SU. Tel: 0181-963 0999. *Fax: 0181-963 1880*

Vitalia Ltd, Paradise, Hemel Hempstead, Herts HP2 4TF. Tel: 01442 231155. *Fax: 01442 218180*

Vitalife Ltd, 291 Cricklewood Lane, London NW2 2JL. Tel: 0181-455 9962. *Fax: 0181-346 0258*

Wallace Manufacturing Chemists, Randles Rd, Knowsley Industrial Park, Merseyside L34 9HX. Tel: 0151-549 1255. *Fax: 0151-549 1064*

Warner-Lambert UK Ltd, (contact Park-Davis Medical), Lambert Court, Chestnut Ave, Eastleigh, Hants SO5 3ZQ. Tel: 01703 620500. *Fax: 01703 629816*

Wassen International Ltd, 14 The Mole Business Park, Leatherhead, Surrey KT22 7BA. Tel: 01372 379828. *Fax: 01372 376599*

Weider Health & Fitness Ltd, Greenroyd Mill, Sutton-in-Craven, Keighley, West Yorkshire BD20 7LW. Tel: 01535 632294. *Fax: 01535 634082*

Whitehall Laboratories Ltd, Huntercombe Lane South, Taplow, Maidenhead, Berkshire SL6 0PH. Tel: 01628 669011 *Fax: 01628 669846*

Windsor Healthcare Ltd, Ellesfield Ave, Bracknell, Berkshire RG12 8YS. Tel 01344 484448. *Fax: 01344 741444*

Index